WORKBOOK FOR DIAGNOSTIC MEDICAL SONOGRAPHY

A Guide to the Vascular System

SECOND EDITION

Rachel Kendoll, BS, MAEd, RVT
Program Director, Vascular Technology
Spokane Community College
Spokane, Washington

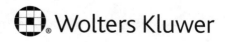 Wolters Kluwer

Philadelphia • Baltimore • New York • London
Buenos Aires • Hong Kong • Sydney • Tokyo

Senior Acquisitions Editor: Sharon Zinner
Development Editor: Amy Millholen
Editorial Coordinator: John Larkin
Marketing Manager: Leah Thomson
Production Project Manager: Kim Cox
Design Coordinator: Joan Wendt
Manufacturing Coordinator: Margie Orzech
Prepress Vendor: S4Carlisle Publishing Services

Second edition

Copyright © 2018 Wolters Kluwer.

9 8 7 6 5 4 3 2

Printed in United States

Library of Congress Cataloging-in-Publication Data

ISBN-13: 978-1-4963-8563-5

ISBN-10: 1-4963-8563-2

Cataloging-in-Publication data available on request from the Publisher.

LWW.com

*To my children, Hannah and Asher—you
are my everything. Thank you for your love
and support—and for sharing me with my
"other kids".
To those "other kids"—my students—you inspire
me to keep learning and persevering everyday.*

*"Around here, we don't look backwards for
very long... We keep moving forward, opening up
new doors and doing new things because
we're curious...and curiosity keeps leading us
down new paths"*
—WALT DISNEY

CONTENTS

PART ONE

FUNDAMENTALS OF ULTRASOUND SCANNING

Orientation to Ultrasound Scanning

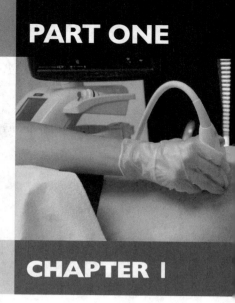

CHAPTER 1

REVIEW OF GLOSSARY TERMS

Matching

Match the key terms with their definitions.

KEY TERMS

1. _____ anechoic

2. _____ coronal plane

3. _____ heterogeneous

4. _____ homogeneous

5. _____ hyperechoic

6. _____ isoechoic

7. _____ sagittal plane

8. _____ transverse plane

DEFINITION

a. A region of an ultrasound image with echoes that are brighter than the surrounding tissue or brighter than normal

b. A vertical plane that divides the body into right and left parts

c. A region of an ultrasound image free from echoes

d. A region of an ultrasound image having mixed or differing ultrasound echoes

e. A plane that divides the body into superior and inferior parts

f. A region of an ultrasound image producing echoes that are the same as the surrounding tissue with equal brightness

g. A region of an ultrasound image having a uniform appearance on ultrasound with echoes that appear similar

h. A vertical plane that divides the body into front and back parts

ANATOMY AND PHYSIOLOGY REVIEW

Image Labeling

Complete the labels in the images that follow.

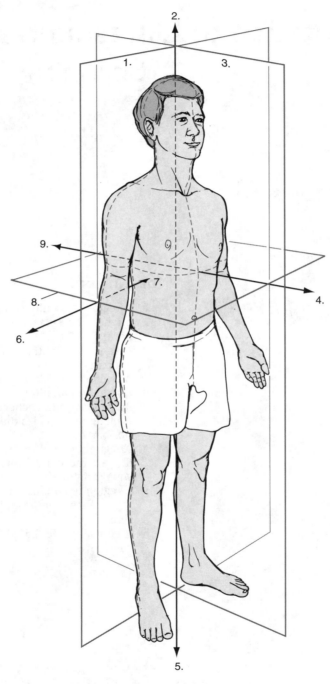

1. Anatomic planes.

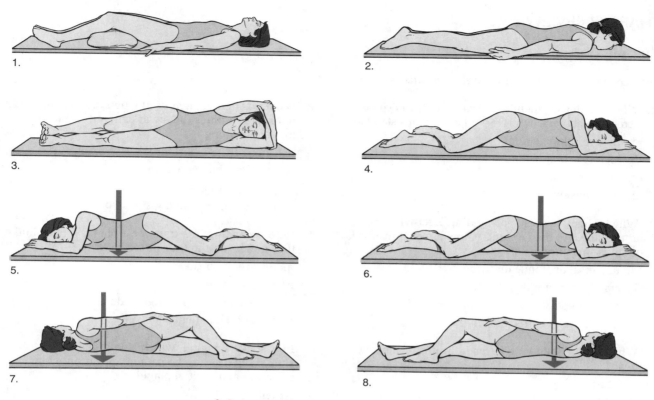

2. Patient positions used in ultrasound scanning.

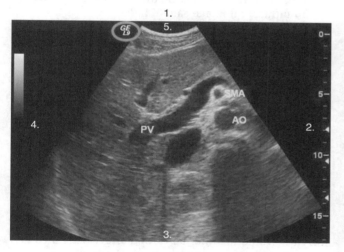

3. Ultrasound image orientation
(label orientation as well as each side of image).

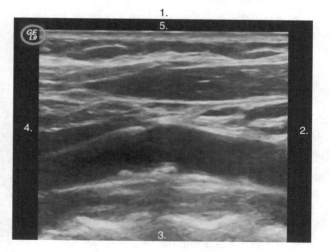

4. Ultrasound image orientation
(label orientation as well as each side of image).

CHAPTER REVIEW

Multiple Choice

Complete each question by circling the best answer.

1. When reading a patient's medical record, you come across the abbreviation HTN. What does this stand for?
   a. hypertrophic nodule
   b. high terminal nephron
   c. hypertension
   d. hypotension

2. When a body is depicted standing erect with arms at the side and the face and palms directed forward, what is this known as?
   a. universal anatomic direction
   b. standard anatomic position
   c. standard positional depiction
   d. anatomically correct position

3. Which of the following terms indicates toward the head?
   a. caudal
   b. posterior
   c. lateral
   d. cephalad

4. Which anatomic plane divides the body into superior and inferior sections?
   a. sagittal
   b. frontal
   c. transverse
   d. coronal

5. If you were to view common carotid artery in long axis, what anatomic body plane would you be using?
   a. sagittal
   b. transverse
   c. coronal
   d. oblique

6. What is a position in which a patient is lying on their left side?
   a. right lateral decubitus
   b. left lateral decubitus
   c. right posterior oblique
   d. left anterior oblique

7. What position would be appropriate if you were to image the right kidney from a posterior approach?
   a. supine
   b. right anterior oblique
   c. prone
   d. right lateral decubitus

8. What position is often used when the vascular technologist examines the lower extremity veins to aid in venous filling?
   a. semi-Fowler's position
   b. Trendelenburg's position
   c. prone position
   d. reverse Trendelenburg's position

9. When scanning in a transverse plane, where should the "notch" on the transducer be?
   a. toward the head
   b. toward the feet
   c. toward the patient's right side
   d. toward the patient's left side

10. In vascular imaging, which side of the screen should the head of the patient appear on when scanning in a sagittal plane?
    a. left
    b. right
    c. top
    d. bottom

11. What is a fluid-filled structure that appears black on an ultrasound image said to be?
    a. hyperechoic
    b. anechoic
    c. echogenic
    d. heterogeneous

12. A mass, which has the same echogenicity as the surrounding liver tissue, is noted within the liver. What term would be used to describe this mass?
    a. isoechoic
    b. hyperechoic
    c. hypoechoic
    d. anechoic

13. How would the internal carotid artery be related directionally to the common carotid artery?
    a. The internal carotid artery is distal to the common carotid artery.
    b. The internal carotid artery is proximal to the common carotid artery.
    c. The internal carotid artery is lateral to the common carotid artery.
    d. The internal carotid artery is medial to the common carotid artery.

14. A patient is discovered to have a blood clot in their leg. What abbreviation would be used for this diagnosis?
    a. CVA
    b. PAD
    c. IDDM
    d. DVT

15. What is a plane that runs vertically through the body but not through the midline?
    a. frontal plane
    b. oblique plane
    c. parasagittal plane
    d. long-axis plane

Fill-in-the-Blank

1. The vertical plane that courses exactly through the midline of the body is the _____ plane.

2. The abbreviation used to describe a stroke would be _____.

3. The coronal plane that splits the body into anterior and posterior sections can also be known as the _____ plane.

4. The transverse plane can also be known as _____ view, especially with reference to viewing a vessel.

5. When imaging the pancreas within the body, the anatomic plane that is typically used is a(n) _____ plane.

6. A good patient position to use to evaluate the spleen would be _____ position.

7. When depicting an image in a transverse plane on an ultrasound image, the left side of the patient should be displayed on the _____ side of the screen.

8. The term used to refer to a structure that produces ultrasound echoes is _____.

9. A plaque noted in the common femoral artery has regions that are anechoic and hyperechoic. This plaque would be described as _____.

10. A directional term that describes a structure that is lower than another structure is _____.

11. The celiac artery would be considered _____, directionally, to the superior mesenteric artery.

12. The abbreviation WNL stands for _____.

13. If the patient is lying supine, medical images are displayed as if viewing the patient from the feet _____.

14. Holding the ultrasound transducer incorrectly can cause the image to be displayed _____.

15. On an ultrasound image, the inner portion of the kidney is brighter than, or _____, when compared to the outer rim of the cortex.

Short Answer

1. Explain the difference between sagittal versus long axis and transverse versus short axis regarding body planes and orientation to the vascular system.

2. Why are appropriate transducer orientation and image standardization important?

IMAGE EVALUATION/PATHOLOGY

Review the images and answer the following questions.

1. Label the imaging planes used to create the images.

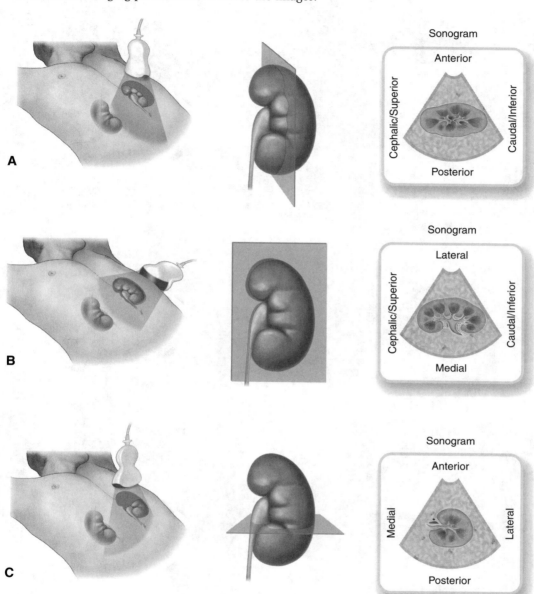

2. Label the patient position and scanning planes used in the images.

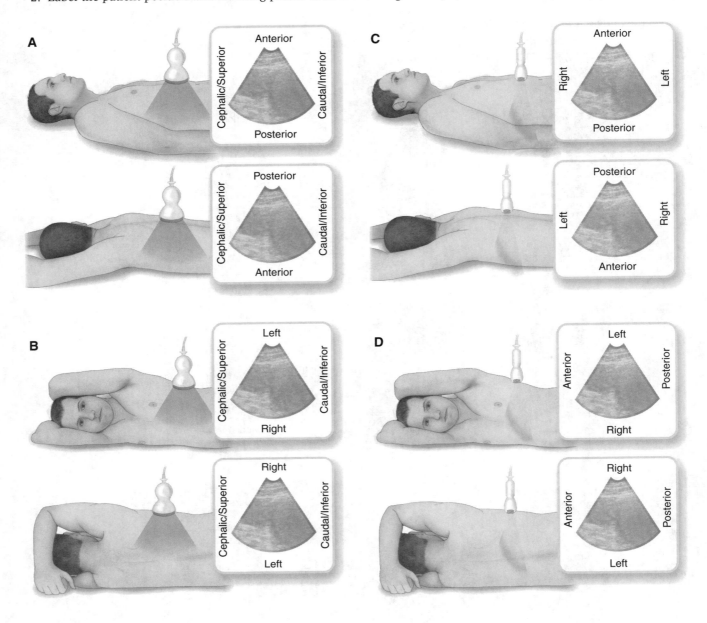

Ultrasound Principles

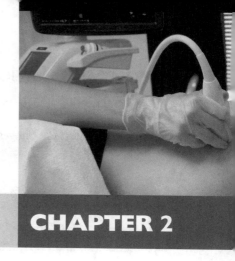

CHAPTER 2

REVIEW OF GLOSSARY TERMS

Matching

Match the key terms with their definitions.

KEY TERMS

1. _____ artifacts

2. _____ bioeffects

3. _____ continuous-wave

4. _____ Doppler

5. _____ pulsed-wave

6. _____ transducer

DEFINITION

a. The part of the ultrasound machine that transmits and receives sound via an array of piezoelectric elements

b. Tool for measuring blood flow quantitatively or qualitatively using pulsed-wave or continuous-wave techniques

c. Echoes on the image not caused by actual reflectors in the body

d. Principle of constantly transmitting a sound wave into the patient to obtain a spectral Doppler waveform

e. The ability of an ultrasound to cause changes to the tissue if proper settings are not used

f. Principle of sending in a small group sound waves and then waiting for the sound to return so that an image can be displayed

ANATOMY AND PHYSIOLOGY REVIEW

Image Labeling

Complete the labels in the images that follow.

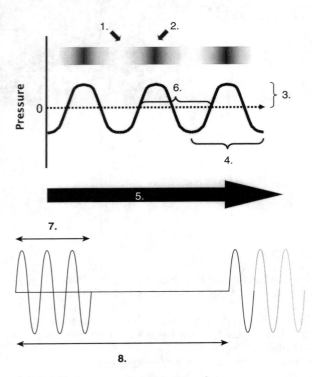

1. Label the wave parameters in these figures.

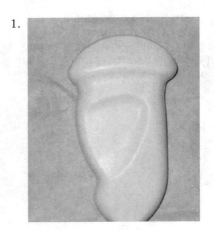

1.

2.

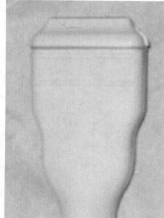

3.

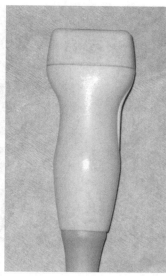

4.

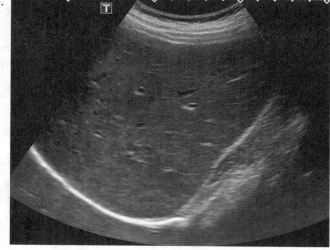

5.

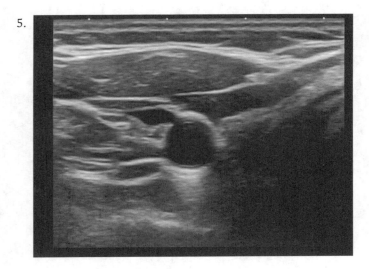

6.

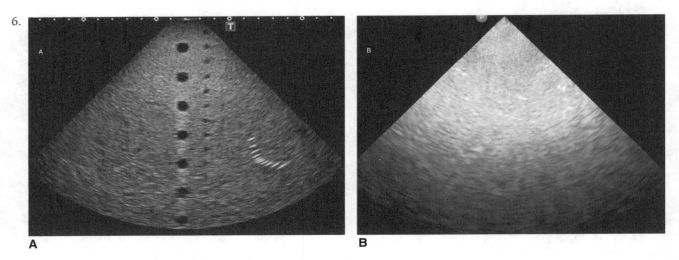

A   B

2. Label these transducers (1–3) and determine which transducer created each image shape (4–6).

CHAPTER REVIEW

Multiple Choice

Complete each question by circling the best answer.

1. What is the number of cycles that occurs in 1 second called?
   a. period
   b. frequency
   c. wavelength
   d. amplitude

2. What is the time taken for one cycle to occur called?
   a. period
   b. frequency
   c. wavelength
   d. propagation speed

3. What determines the propagation speed of sound?
   a. the source of the sound
   b. the thickness of the piezoelectric crystal
   c. the medium through which the sound is moving
   d. both the sound source and the medium

4. What is the height of a cycle from baseline to the peak of the cycle called?
   a. frequency
   b. propagation speed
   c. acoustic impedance
   d. amplitude

5. What is the number of pulses per second emitted by an ultrasound system called?
   a. spatial pulse length
   b. pulse repetition frequency
   c. pulse repetition period
   d. pulse duration

6. What information is needed in order to determine spatial pulse length?
   a. frequency and wavelength
   b. propagation speed and the number of cycles per pulse
   c. wavelength and the number of cycles per pulse
   d. period and pulse repetition frequency

7. What is the percentage of time the machine is transmitting sound in to the patient called?
   a. pulse repetition period
   b. duty factor
   c. acoustic impedance
   d. frame rate

8. What is the minimum number of piezoelectric elements necessary to perform continuous-wave Doppler?
   a. one
   b. two
   c. three
   d. ten

9. Which of the following has the highest attenuation?
   a. water
   b. muscle
   c. bone
   d. air

10. What type of reflection results when sound encounters structures that are smaller than the transmitted beam's wavelength?
    a. specular
    b. nonspecular
    c. refractory
    d. Rayleigh scattering

11. Which of the following must be present for reflection to occur?
    a. acoustic impedance mismatch
    b. difference in propagation speeds between two media
    c. structures much smaller than the ultrasound beam's wavelength
    d. a change in the direction of the sound beam

12. What is a change in direction of the transmitted beam at an interface called?
    a. reflection
    b. backscatter
    c. refraction
    d. attenuation

13. Assuming soft tissue, how long does it take an ultrasound pulse to reach a depth of 1 cm and return to the transducer?
    a. 6.5 µs
    b. 13 µs
    c. 26 µs
    d. 1,540 m/s

14. Which transducer is most commonly used for peripheral and cerebrovascular examinations?
    a. curvilinear array
    b. linear sequential array
    c. phased array
    d. annular array

15. Which transducer creates a "pie slice" shaped image?
    a. curvilinear array
    b. linear sequential array
    c. phased array
    d. annular array

16. Which of the following is added to a transducer to limit the number of cycles in a pulse?
    a. damping material
    b. matching layer
    c. attenuation layer
    d. lead zirconate titanate

17. After removing gel and fluids from a non-intracavitary transducer, what should be the next step in cleaning the transducer?
    a. Apply sterile probe cover.
    b. Submerge in high-level disinfectant.
    c. Wipe down with low-level disinfectant.
    d. Sterilize by autoclave.

18. What is the part of the ultrasound machine that provides the electricity that shocks the transducer called?
    a. attenuator
    b. receiver
    c. damping material
    d. pulser

19. What does the acronym ALARA stand for?
    a. as low as reasonably achievable
    b. as light as reference allows
    c. apply low-amplitude reflector attenuators
    d. as low as reflection allows

20. What does the TI indicate?
    a. risk of mechanical bioeffects
    b. risk of attenuation
    c. risk of thermal bioeffects
    d. measure of the beam's intensity

21. Which plane describes the resolution parallel to the beam?
    a. temporal
    b. axial
    c. lateral
    d. transverse

22. Where is the lateral resolution the best?
    a. focal zone
    b. near field
    c. far field
    d. divergent zone

23. A reflector moving toward a transducer would result in what type of Doppler shift?
    a. negative shift
    b. positive shift
    c. zero shift
    d. maximum shift

24. What angle results in the most accurate and highest Doppler shift?
    a. 0 degrees
    b. 60 degrees
    c. 90 degrees
    d. any angle between 45 and 60 degrees

25. On a spectral display, what is represented on the vertical axis?
    a. time
    b. velocity
    c. signal amplitude
    d. depth

26. How is the Nyquist limit calculated?
    a. ¼ PRF
    b. 2× PRF
    c. 4× PRF
    d. ½ PRF

27. What is a complex processing technique that converts complex frequency shifts into a spectral waveform?
    a. fast Fourier transform
    b. spectral broadening
    c. autocorrelation
    d. Nyquist criterion

28. Which of the following describes sending multiple pulses down one scan line to create a color Doppler image?
    a. Nyquist criterion
    b. ensemble length
    c. autocorrelation
    d. fast Fourier transform

29. What is a Doppler technique that provides flow information based on amplitude of the Doppler shift, not the shift itself?
    a. color Doppler
    b. CW Doppler
    c. spectral Doppler
    d. power Doppler

30. Which control adjusts the overall brightness of the B-mode image?
    a. TGC
    b. compression
    c. gain
    d. frequency

31. Which processing technique results in better lateral resolution and reduces reverberation artifact?
    a. spatial compounding
    b. tissue harmonic imaging
    c. time gain compensation
    d. fast Fourier transform

32. Which control should be adjusted to permit the display of higher velocities in a spectral Doppler display?
    a. spectral gain
    b. PRF/Scale
    c. angle correction
    d. sweep speed

33. Which control should be adjusted if color is either not filling the vessel or is bleeding outside the vessel wall?
    a. color invert
    b. color gate size
    c. color gain
    d. color frequency

34. During an ultrasound evaluation of the aorta, a surgical clip is encountered. What artifact would likely be present owing to this clip?
    a. shadowing
    b. comet tail
    c. enhancement
    d. mirror image

35. What is an artifact caused by wall motion that can be reduced by using a wall filter?
    a. clutter
    b. mirror image
    c. reverberation
    d. grating lobes

Fill-in-the-Blank

1. Sound waves are _____, indicating that the movement of the molecules within the wave is parallel to propagation direction.

2. The typically frequency range used in medical diagnostic ultrasound is _____ MHz.

3. The average propagation speed in soft tissue that ultrasound machines use is _____ m/s.

4. The property of the medium that is determined by the product of the density and propagation speed that helps determine reflection of echoes is _____.

5. The parameter that primarily determines pulse repetition frequency and period is _____.

6. The loss of some energy in the sound beam as it travels through tissue is _____.

7. The average rate of attenuation through soft tissue is _____.

8. The diaphragm is an example of a _____ reflector.

9. A red blood cell is an example of a _____ scatterer.

10. If the propagation speed in the second medium is greater than 1,540 m/s, the angle of the transmitted beam will be _____ than the incident angle.

11. The ultrasound machine uses the _____ equation to determine the travel time of an ultrasound pulse.

12. Modern transducers are _____, meaning they have the ability to use different frequencies that are present in the beam.

13. The _____ layer of a transducer is used to improve transmission of sound into the patient.

14. The piezoelectric elements within a transducer are usually made of _____.

15. The measure of the amount of power in an ultrasound beam divided by the area of the beam is the _____.

16. A bioeffect of ultrasound that results in the creation of bubbles in the tissue is _____.

17. No bioeffects have been noted with an unfocused transducer with an intensity below _____ mW/cm^2.

18. Lateral resolution is determined by the _____ of the beam.

19. Axial resolution is improved by increasing the _____ of the transducer.

20. The number of images produced per second is called the _____.

21. The _____ is the difference between the transmitted frequency of the ultrasound transducer and the returned frequency of the reflector.

22. A Doppler angle of _____ degrees results in no detectable shift.

23. A common artifact of PW spectral Doppler is _____, or wraparound of the spectral waveform causing positive shifts to be displayed as negative.

24. The maximum frequency shift that can be sampled during PW Doppler is known as the _____.

25. Filling in of the spectral window because of a wide range of velocities at a given point in time is called _____.

26. The process used in color Doppler to identify mean velocity and direction is called _____.

27. Slider controls used to achieve uniform brightness across an image are known as _____.

28. A processing technique that sends the beam into the patient from different directions to improve the appearance of soft tissue is known as _____.

29. A Doppler control that allows the display of more or fewer spectral waveforms on the screen at one time is _____.

30. _____ artifact occurs as a result of attenuation of sound and is often seen posterior to bone or calcified plaque.

Short Answer

1. Why are air and bone best avoided during an ultrasound exam?

2. What is the piezoelectric effect?

3. What are the appropriate steps to clean and disinfect an ultrasound transducer?

4. What are some measures a sonographer can take to follow the ALARA principle?

5. What factors determine and affect temporal resolution?

IMAGE EVALUATION/PATHOLOGY

Review the images and answer the following questions.

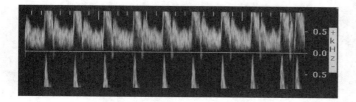

1. a. What artifact is being displayed in this image?
   b. What can be done to correct this artifact?

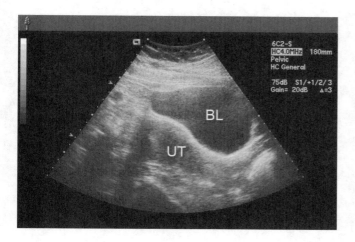

2. What artifact is being displayed in this image?

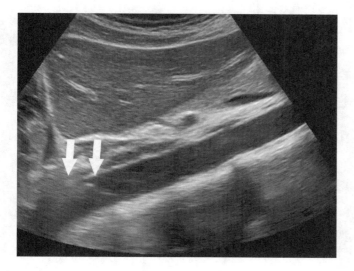

3. What artifact is being displayed in this image?

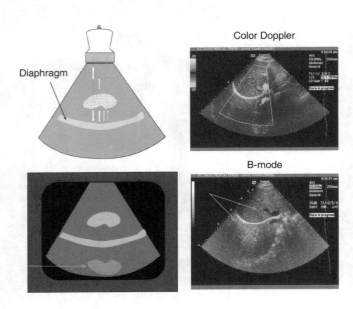

Diaphragm

Color Doppler

B-mode

4. What artifact is being displayed in this image?

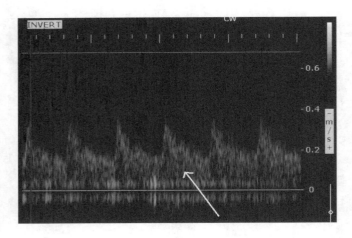

5. What artifact is being displayed in this image?

Ergonomics: Avoiding Work-Related Injury

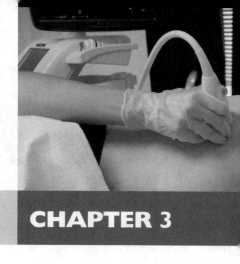

CHAPTER 3

REVIEW OF GLOSSARY TERMS

Matching

Match the key terms with their definitions.

KEY TERMS

1. _____ awkward postures

2. _____ contact stress

3. _____ duration

4. _____ force

5. _____ load/loading

6. _____ repetition

7. _____ static postures

DEFINITION

a. Period of time that a body part is exposed to an ergonomic risk factor

b. Situation when body parts are positioned away from their neutral position

c. The force exerted by an object on a contracted muscle

d. Situation when a body part is held in a single position over a long period of time

e. Sustained contact between a body part and an external object

f. Repeated motion that includes other ergonomic risk factors, such as force and/or awkward posture

g. The exertion of physical effort applied by a body part to perform a task

CHAPTER REVIEW

Multiple Choice

Complete each question by circling the best answer.

1. At what age do work-related musculoskeletal disorders generally peak?
   a. 55 to 64
   b. 65 to 75
   c. 45 to 54
   d. 30 to 40

2. What causes most work-related musculoskeletal disorders?
   a. single, initiating injury or exposure to risk factor
   b. repeated exposure to one or more risk factors
   c. initial injury followed by secondary similar injury
   d. maintaining neutral postures during exam performance

3. Which of the following are risk factors for the development of WRMSDs?
   a. exerting excessive force
   b. contact pressure of a body part
   c. vibration
   d. all of the above

4. What is the most commonly reported symptom reported by sonographers?
   a. low back pain
   b. hand and wrist pain
   c. shoulder pain
   d. neck pain

5. According to the 1997 Health Care Benefit Trust study, what percentage of sonographers reported musculoskeletal pain related to scanning?
   a. 71%
   b. 81%
   c. 90%
   d. 54%

6. What is a major result of repeated exposure to risk factors for WRMSDs?
   a. Interference with the ability of the body to recover
   b. Acute onset of initial injury
   c. Sudden onset of symptoms related to exposure
   d. Rapid disease progression and musculoskeletal deterioration

7. Which condition results in compression of nerves and deterioration of tendons and ligaments?
   a. microtears
   b. degeneration
   c. inflammation
   d. swelling

8. What is the by-product of muscle metabolism that, when built up, results in pain?
   a. lactic acid
   b. hydrochloric acid
   c. lactose
   d. mitochondrial acid

9. Which of the following results from friction between a tendon and its sheath, resulting in inflammation and swelling of the tendon?
   a. tendonitis
   b. tenosynovitis
   c. bursitis
   d. epicondylitis

10. What can result when an inflamed tendon sheath fills with lubricating fluid, causing a bump under the skin?
    a. carpal tunnel syndrome
    b. epicondylitis
    c. Ganglion cyst
    d. tensynovitis

11. What can result when a tendon attempts to bear the load usually required of a muscle?
    a. tendonitis
    b. tenosynovitis
    c. bursitis
    d. epicondylitis

12. What percentage of sonographers who were symptomatic for WRMSDs suffered career-ending injuries?
    a. 81%
    b. 54%
    c. 33%
    d. 20%

13. What is the type of posture that requires the least amount of muscular effort, protecting muscles and tendons from injury?
    a. non-neutral posture
    b. awkward posture
    c. neutral posture
    d. neural posture

14. During performance of an ultrasound examination, under what degree of abduction should the sonographer keep their scanning arm?
    a. 10 degrees
    b. 20 degrees
    c. 30 degrees
    d. 40 degrees

15. When adjusting the monitor of the ultrasound system, to what level should the monitor be positioned?
    a. chin level
    b. eye level
    c. as low as possible
    d. above the sonographer's head

16. What type of grip would be best to use when holding the transducer?
    a. palmar grip
    b. pinch grip
    c. tight grip
    d. force grip

17. What regulatory agency determines the laws and requirements that employers must follow regarding workplace safety?
    a. WRMSD
    b. WRSHA
    c. OSHA
    d. ACLU

18. Which equipment piece should be adjusted throughout the ultrasound examination?
    a. chair
    b. table
    c. ultrasound machine
    d. all of the above

19. When performing an ultrasound examination on a difficult to image patient (high BMI, limited mobility), the sonographer should do all of the following EXCEPT:
    a. limit time during the exam to minimize exposure to WRMSD risk factors.
    b. use correct body mechanics throughout as much as possible.
    c. push as hard as possible throughout the entire exam using a forceful grip on the transducer.
    d. accept any limitations of the imaging capabilities for the exam.

20. What adjustment do most sonographers NOT do with the exam table during an ultrasound examination?
    a. Raise it high enough to limit reaching.
    b. Lower it enough to minimize arm abduction.
    c. Move it close enough to the ultrasound machine to prevent falls.
    d. Lock the wheels to prevent movement during the exam.

Fill-in-the-Blank

1. _____ is defined as painful conditions that are caused or aggravated by workplace activities.

2. Despite many improvements in ergonomic equipment and training, a 2009 study reported that _____% of clinical sonographers reported symptoms of WRMSDs, an increase from the 1997 study.

3. Many tasks contribute to WRMSDs, including physical, psychosocial, and _____ work practices.

4. Risk factors and injuries related to WRMSDs may not be readily apparent as symptoms occur after _____.

5. Awkward postures often lead to restriction of blood flow into contracted muscles as a result of _____ on the blood vessels.

6. Recovery time is important to muscle function because it allows the muscles to relax and for _____ to be flushed out.

7. The general term for inflammation of the tendon, usually as a result of repeated stress causing tendon fibers to tear, is _____.

8. A sac of lubricating fluid that is present in a joint where tendons pass through a narrow space between bones is known as a _____.

9. Inflammation can result in nerve _____, causing weakness, tingling sensations, and numbness.

10. From the standpoint of prevention of WRMSDs, it is better to _____ the ultrasound system during transport rather than _____ it.

11. Symptoms of WRMSDs may be present at _____, after prolonged exposure to risks rather than while performing work tasks.

12. One of the most prevalent risk factors for sonographers is _____, which requires excess muscle firing and a quicker onset of fatigue.

13. When performing an ultrasound examination, the ultrasound system should be positioned _____ to the exam table, with no appreciable space between the two.

14. Elbow flexion of either the scanning or nonscanning arm should be _____ degrees or more.

15. When using a chair, the height should be adjusted to maintain a neutral trunk, neck, and arm posture and ensure that the knees are slightly _____ than the hips.

16. During a sonographic procedure, the patient should be positioned at the _____ edge of the exam table to reduce abduction and reach.

17. Providing an external _____ for the patient to observe can prevent twisting of the neck and back of the sonographer.

18. Not only should the ultrasound examination room and equipment be adjusted ergonomically, the _____ workstation used for PACS or electronic medical records entry should be adjustable as well.

19. A simple modification to reduce strain and fatigue of the shoulder and neck muscles is to support the scanning arm using _____ or a _____ under the elbow.

20. Employer and academic programs as well as professional organizations provide options for ongoing _____ and _____ regarding proper scanning techniques and avoiding work-related injuries.

Short Answer

1. What psychosocial risk factors contribute to WRMSDs?

2. What factors and tasks, including those not directly related to performance of a sonographic exam, contribute to WRMSDs?

3. What are some examples of the concept of "large before small"?

4. Why is recognition of symptoms and early reporting and treatment of WRMSDs important?

5. What are the components of the neutral scanning posture recommended for sonographers to avoid WRMSDs?

CASE STUDY

1. You are asked to consult with another sonographer regarding scanning more ergonomically. When you observe the sonographer, you notice many awkward postures are being used and the ultrasound system, chair, and table all need adjusted. What advice would you give this sonographer to resolve the awkward postures and adjust the equipment?

PART TWO

INTRODUCTION TO THE VASCULAR SYSTEM

Vascular Anatomy

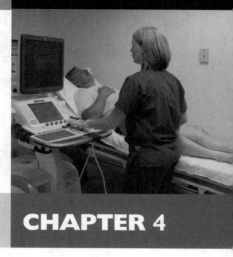

CHAPTER 4

REVIEW OF GLOSSARY TERMS

Matching

Match the key terms with their definitions.

KEY TERMS

1. _____ artery

2. _____ arteriole

3. _____ capillary

4. _____ venule

5. _____ vein

DEFINITION

a. A small blood vessel with only endothelium and basement membrane through which exchange of nutrients and waste occurs
b. A small vein that is continuous with a capillary
c. A blood vessel that carries blood away from the heart
d. A small artery with a muscular wall; a terminal artery, which continues into the capillary network
e. A blood vessel that carries blood toward the heart

ANATOMY AND PHYSIOLOGY REVIEW

Image Labeling

Complete the labels in the images that follow.

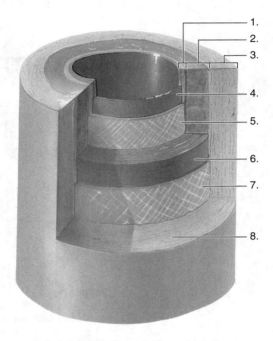

1. _____
2. _____
3. _____
4. _____
5. _____
6. _____
7. _____
8. _____

1. Schematic diagram of arterial walls.

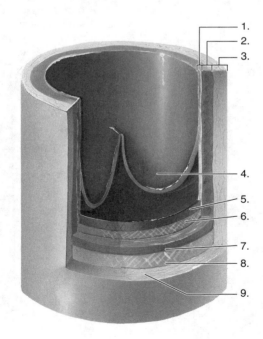

1. _____
2. _____
3. _____
4. _____
5. _____
6. _____
7. _____
8. _____
9. _____

2. Schematic diagram of venous walls.

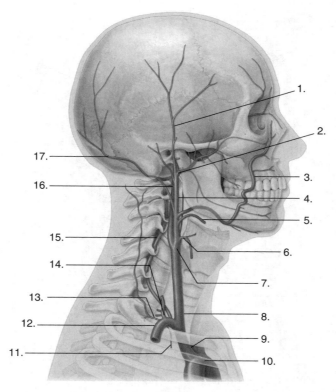

3. Illustration of the external carotid artery and its branches.

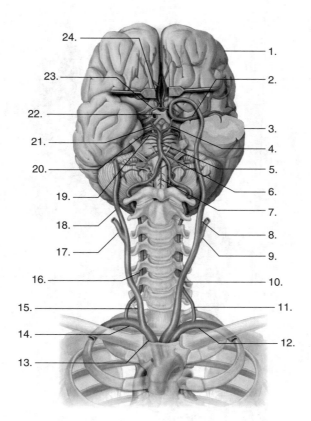

4. Diagram indicating the orientation of the vertebral arteries through the cervical vertebrae and into the cranial cavity.

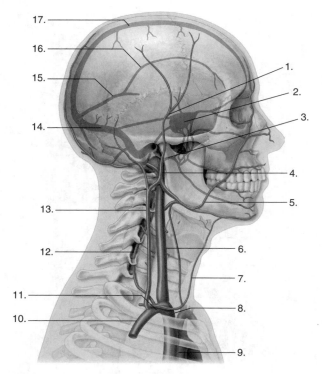

5. Venous drainage of the brain, head, and neck.

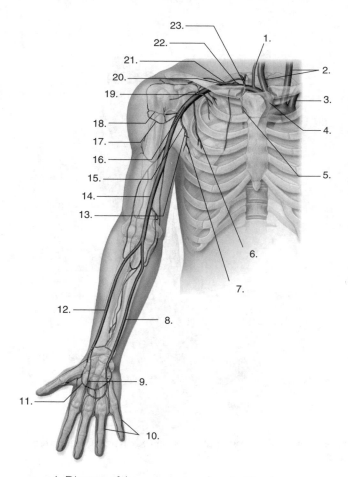

6. Diagram of the upper extremity arterial system.

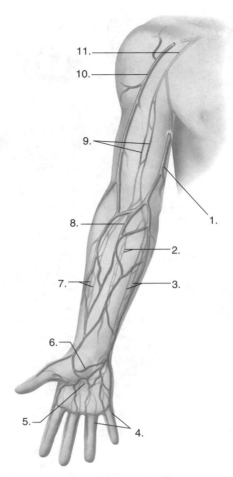

7. Venous drainage of the hand and veins of the upper extremity.

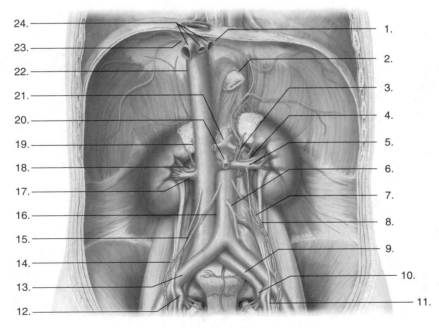

8. The abdominal aorta and its branches, as well as inferior vena cava and its tributaries.

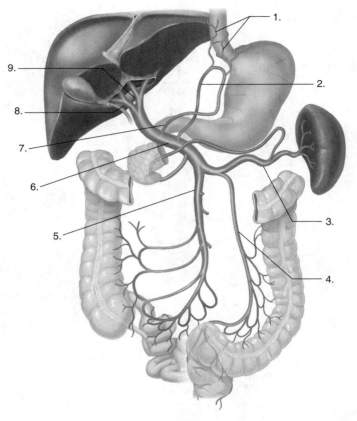

9. Diagram illustrating the main portal vein and its tributaries.

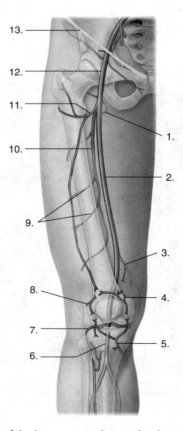

10. Diagram of the lower extremity arteries through the thigh.

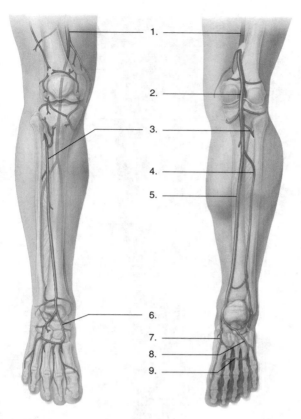

11. Diagram of the lower extremity arteries through the calf.

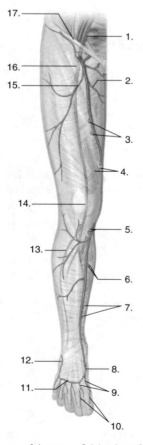

12. Diagram of the superficial veins of the leg.

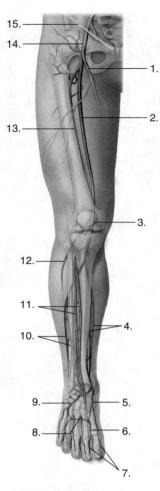

13. Diagram of the lower extremity deep venous system.

CHAPTER REVIEW

Multiple Choice

Complete each question by circling the best answer.

1. At which level of the circulatory system does exchange of oxygen, carbon dioxide, waste, and nutrients occur?
   a. aorta
   b. inferior vena cava
   c. arterioles
   d. capillaries

2. Which statement describes the exchange of nutrients and oxygen at the level of the capillaries?
   a. Carbon dioxide and waste reabsorption takes place in the venules.
   b. Nutrient and oxygen exchange is simultaneous to carbon dioxide and waste exchange.
   c. Nutrients and oxygen exchange occurs at the venous side only.
   d. Capillary permeability for nutrient and oxygen exchange is the same within all tissue beds.

3. Which statement describes capillary permeability to large molecules?
   a. It is the same in all tissues.
   b. It varies depending on the characteristics of the tissue bed.
   c. It only varies with the tissue beds in the brain.
   d. It is selective only in the liver.

4. Why can arterioles control the resistance of the vascular bed?
   a. They have concentric layers of smooth muscle cells.
   b. They are the smallest arteries in the circulatory system.
   c. They are the vessels leading to the capillaries.
   d. They have all three main layers of tissue: intima, media, and adventitia.

5. Which of the following is NOT an example of a large elastic artery?

   a. the common carotid arteries

   b. the superficial femoral arteries

   c. the common iliac arteries

   d. the aorta

6. What is the main difference between arteries and veins of a similar size in regard to the composition of their walls?

   a. Veins have thinner walls overall with less muscle.

   b. Veins have thicker walls with more elastic fibers.

   c. Veins have thinner walls overall with more muscle.

   d. Arteries have thinner walls overall with more muscle.

7. Which of the following is NOT an example of a large vein?

   a. the portal vein

   b. the inferior vena cava

   c. the superior vena cava

   d. the brachial vein

8. Which statement regarding venous valves is FALSE?

   a. They allow for bidirectional flow under normal conditions.

   b. They are more numerous in the veins of the lower extremities.

   c. They are usually absent from veins in the thorax and abdomen.

   d. They have only two leaflets.

9. What structure forms venous valves?

   a. three semilunar cusps

   b. the elastic and collagen fibers from the basement membrane

   c. projections of the intima layer

   d. projections of the media layer

10. Which statement regarding the first branch of the internal carotid artery is TRUE?

   a. The ophthalmic artery is usually the first branch at the petrous level.

   b. The ophthalmic artery is usually the first branch at the cavernous level.

   c. The ophthalmic artery is usually the first branch at the cerebral level.

   d. The internal carotid artery does not have branches.

11. From where does the left common carotid artery typically arise?

   a. the left subclavian artery

   b. the aortic arch

   c. the innominate artery

   d. the right subclavian artery

12. Which statement regarding the venous drainage of the head and neck is FALSE?

   a. Drainage occurs in the posterior portion via vertebral veins.

   b. Vertebral veins are formed by a dense venous plexus.

   c. The external jugular veins drain into the brachiocephalic veins.

   d. The internal jugular veins drain into the brachiocephalic veins.

13. Which tissues do branches of the right or left subclavian arteries supply?

   a. the brain and neck

   b. the thoracic wall and shoulder

   c. the aortic arch

   d. both A and B

14. Which artery is NOT typically a branch of the ulnar arteries?

   a. the radial artery

   b. the interosseous artery

   c. the recurrent ulnar artery

   d. the superficial palmar arch

15. Which of the following is NOT a superficial vein of the upper extremities?

   a. the interosseous veins

   b. the basilic veins

   c. the cephalic veins

   d. the medial antebrachial veins

16. What are the three branches of the celiac trunk or celiac artery?

   a. the SMA, IMA, and hepatic artery

   b. the SMA, right gastric artery, and left gastric artery

   c. the splenic, left gastric, and hepatic arteries

   d. the splenic, right gastric, and hepatic arteries

17. What is another name for the internal iliac arteries?

   a. the hypergastric arteries

   b. the hypogastric arteries

   c. the epigastric arteries

   d. the subgastric arteries

18. Which of the following are the terminal branches of the popliteal artery?

   a. the tibial and peroneal arteries

   b. the genicular and sural arteries

   c. the anterior and posterior tibial arteries

   d. the anterior tibial artery and tibioperoneal trunk

19. Where does the deep venous system of the lower extremities start?
    a. the deep plantar arch
    b. the medial plantar arch
    c. the lateral plantar arch
    d. the dorsal venous arch

20. Typically, what happens as the popliteal vein and artery pass through the adductor canal?
    a. The vein moves from medial to lateral of the artery.
    b. The vein moves from lateral to medial of the artery.
    c. The vein moves from anterior to posterior of the artery.
    d. The vein moves from posterior to anterior of the artery.

Fill-in-the-Blank

1. Exchange of gasses, nutrients, and wastes occurs mainly at the level of _____ in the circulatory system.

2. The venous side of the capillaries is drained by _____.

3. Arterioles are the main control of _____ of the circulatory system.

4. Arteries are classified not only according to size but also in the composition of the _____.

5. The femoral arteries, the brachial arteries, and the mesenteric arteries are examples of _____.

6. Lower extremity veins have _____ walls than upper extremity veins.

7. The thickest layer in large veins is _____.

8. The bulk of the wall composition in large veins is an adventitia that contains _____.

9. The valves found in veins are called _____ because they have two semilunar leaflets.

10. The petrous, cavernous, and cerebral levels correspond to the _____ portion of the internal carotid artery.

11. A unique arrangement of the intracranial branches of the internal carotid and vertebral arteries serving as an important collateral network is called _____.

12. The first and largest branch of the aortic arch is the _____.

13. Typically, the _____ is considered the first and largest branch of the brachial artery.

14. The upper extremity superficial vein coursing along the medial border of the biceps muscle is the _____.

15. The bronchial, esophageal, phrenic, intercostal, and subcostal arteries are branches of the _____.

16. Two branches of the anterior-lateral surface of the aorta just below the level of the renal arteries are the _____.

17. The right and left common iliac arteries bifurcate from the abdominal aorta, typically at the level of the _____.

18. Another name of the deep femoral artery is _____.

19. The continuation of the lateral segment of the dorsal venous arch is _____.

20. The veins that pass between the tibia and fibula through the upper part of the interosseous membrane are the _____.

Short Answer

1. Why have arterioles been called the stopcocks of the circulatory system?

2. What are the major differences in wall composition between arteries and veins?

3. Describe how the popliteal artery divides into the various calf vessels and how the veins are configured out of the calf back to the popliteal vein.

4. The liver has a unique arrangement of vessels and receives blood from two sources. What are the two sources?

5. Where do the deep and superficial venous systems originate in the lower extremity?

IMAGE EVALUATION/PATHOLOGY

Review the images and answer the following questions.

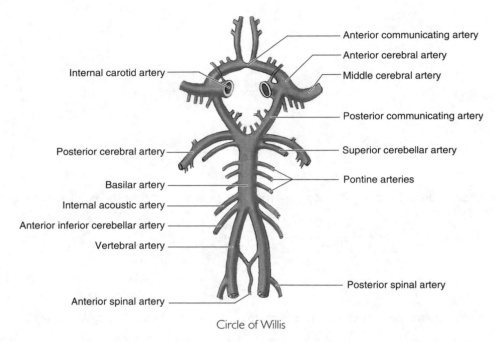

Circle of Willis

1. Using this figure as a guide, describe a collateral pathway that could be used to perfuse the brain if the left internal carotid artery was occluded.

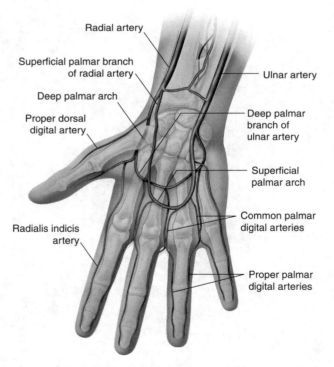

Radial artery supplying the deep palmar arch

2. A common procedure in cardiovascular surgery is to use the radial artery as a conduit for coronary artery bypass grafting. Using this figure as a guide, describe how the hand would remain perfused if the radial artery was harvested for this procedure.

Arterial Physiology

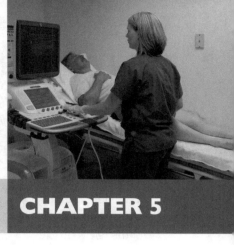

CHAPTER 5

REVIEW OF GLOSSARY TERMS

Matching

Match the key terms with their definitions.

KEY TERMS

1. _B_ potential energy

2. _A_ kinetic energy

3. _D_ Poiseuille's law

4. _C_ laminar flow

5. _F_ viscosity

6. _E_ inertia

DEFINITION

a. The energy of work or motion; in the vascular system, it is in part represented by the velocity of blood flow

b. The stored or resting energy; in the vascular system, it is the intravascular pressure

c. Flow of a liquid in which it travels smoothly in parallel layers

d. The law that states the volume flow of a liquid flowing through a vessel is directly proportional to the pressure of the liquid and the fourth power of the radius and is inversely proportional to the viscosity of the liquid and the length of the vessel

e. The tendency of a body at rest to stay at rest or a body in motion to stay in motion

f. The property of a fluid that resists the force tending to cause fluid to flow

CHAPTER REVIEW

Multiple Choice

Complete each question by circling the best answer.

1. Where in the vascular system is the lowest energy represented by the lowest pressure located?
   a. the right atrium
   b. the left atrium
   c. the right ventricle
   d. the left ventricle

2. Which of the following statements regarding the gravitational energy and hydrostatic pressure is FALSE?
   a. They are components of the total energy in the vascular system.
   b. They tend to cancel each other.
   c. They are components of the kinetic energy in the vascular system.
   d. They are expressed in relation to a reference point.

3. What causes blood in the vascular system to move from one point to the next?
   a. hydraulic filtering
   b. pressure or energy gradient
   c. hydrostatic pressure
   d. inertia

4. In the entire vascular system, how does the cross-sectional area of vessels change?
   a. Increases from the aorta to the capillary level.
   b. Decreases from the aorta to the capillary level.
   c. Remains the same from the aorta to the capillary level.
   d. Increases only at the level of the arterioles.

5. Which of the following statements regarding the velocity of the blood flow is FALSE?
   a. Velocity refers to the rate of displacement of blood in time.
   b. The velocity of the blood increases from the capillaries to the venous system.
   c. The velocity of the blood increases from the aorta to the capillaries.
   d. The velocity of the blood changes with cross-sectional area of the vessels.

6. Which of the following could NOT be used as a unit to measure flow volume?
   a. mL/s
   b. m/s
   c. cL/min
   d. L/min

7. In the vascular system, what represents the potential difference or voltage in Ohm's law?
   a. volume flow
   b. resistance
   c. pressure gradient
   d. vessel radius

8. Changes in which of the following will most significantly affect resistance in the vascular system?
   a. volume flow
   b. velocity
   c. viscosity of the blood
   d. radius of vessels

9. When vessels are arranged in parallel, how does this affect the entire system?
   a. lower total resistance than when vessels are in series
   b. higher total resistance than when vessels are in series
   c. does not affect the total resistance of a system
   d. disrupts flow in collaterals

10. Which of the following characterizes low-resistance flow?
    a. retrograde flow
    b. alternating antegrade/retrograde flow
    c. antegrade flow
    d. constriction of arteriolar bed

11. Which of the following characteristics regarding high-resistance flow is FALSE?
    a. The flow profile may be two to three phases.
    b. The flow displays alternating antegrade/retrograde flow.
    c. The flow profile is due to vasoconstriction of arterioles.
    d. The flow profile is due to vasodilation of arterioles.

12. What flow profile is typically demonstrated at the entrance of a vessel?
    a. plug flow
    b. laminar flow
    c. turbulent flow
    d. streamlined flow

13. Which of the following statements regarding laminar flow is FALSE?
    a. The layers of cells at the center of the vessels move the fastest.
    b. The layers of cells at the wall of the vessels do not move.
    c. The velocity at the center of the vessels is half the mean velocity.
    d. The difference in velocities between layers is due to friction.

14. What is required to move blood flow in a turbulent system?
    a. higher velocities
    b. greater pressure
    c. larger radius
    d. smaller radius

15. What is the function of the hydraulic filter of the arterial system (composed of the elastic arteries and high-resistance arterioles)?
    a. Ensure adequate gas/nutrient exchange in the arteries.
    b. Convert the cardiac output flow to steady flow.
    c. Ensure adequate conduction of the pressure wave.
    d. Distribute flow to the capillaries.

16. In diastole, how is the conversion of potential energy into blood flow accomplished?
    a. ejection of the stroke volume from the heart
    b. elastic recoil of the arteries
    c. cardiac contraction
    d. hydraulic filtering effect

17. How is the resistance in the arterial system controlled?
    a. By the contraction and relaxation of smooth muscle cells in the media of arterioles.
    b. By the contraction and relaxation of the heart.
    c. By the contraction and relaxation of muscle cells in the surrounding tissue.
    d. By the capacitance of the arterial system.

18. Which of the following will result when norepinephrine is released by the sympathetic nervous system?
    a. The relaxation of smooth muscle cells in arterioles is triggered
    b. The contraction of smooth muscle cells in arterioles is triggered
    c. No effect on the smooth muscle cells in arterioles
    d. No effect on the tone of the arteriole walls

19. Most prominently, abnormal energy losses in the arterial system would result from pathologies such as obstruction and/or stenoses because of which of the following?
    a. the increased length of the stenosis
    b. the friction from the atherosclerotic plaque
    c. the decrease in the vessel's radius
    d. the increased viscosity

20. Which of the following statements about collateral vessels is FALSE?
    a. Collaterals are preexisting pathways.
    b. The resistance in collaterals is mostly fixed.
    c. Vasodilator drugs have a large effect on collaterals.
    d. Midzone collaterals are small intramuscular branches.

Fill-in-the-Blank

1. In the human body, the major component of the blood influencing viscosity is _hematocrit_

2. The highest pressure in the vascular system (of approximately 120 mm Hg) is found in the _Left ventricle_

3. When moving farther from the reference point of the right atrium, the hydrostatic pressure _increases_.

4. The principle stating that the total energy remains constant from one point to another without changes in flow velocity is _Bernouli's principle_

5. Inertia and viscosity are two components of the vascular system contributing to _energy loss_

6. In the vascular system, if the volume of blood or flow remains the same, a decrease in the area of a vessel should trigger a(n) _increase_ in the velocity of blood.

7. The law defined by the statement that the current through two points is directly proportional to the potential difference across the two points and inversely proportional to the resistance between them is _Ohm's law_.

8. The total resistance in a system where the elements are arranged in series is the _Sum_ of the individual resistances.

9. A low-resistance flow profile characteristically displays _antegrade_ flow throughout the cardiac cycle.

10. The third antegrade phase seen in a high-resistance flow profile is related to _Compliance_ of the proximal vessels.

11. After exercise, under normal conditions, the resistance of the tissue bed in the lower extremities will change from _high to low_

12. In laminar flow, the "layers" of cells at the center of the vessel move _faster_ than the layers closest to the wall of the vessel.

13. Turbulence in a blood vessel is mostly the result of change in the velocity of blood and the _radius_ of the vessel.

14. The Reynolds number above which turbulence of flow starts to occur is _2000_.

15. The arterial system can be compared to the _hydraulic filter_ of the resistance–capacitance filters of an electrical circuit.

16. Pulse pressure in the arterial system is the difference between _systolic_ and _diastolic_ pressure.

17. An example of a local feedback mechanism that controls blood flow is that a drop in interstitial _oxygen_ will trigger the arterioles to dilate.

18. In an area of atherosclerotic plaque, the exposure of the subendothelial collagen matrix is _thrombogenic_ and may cause platelet accumulation.

19. Energy losses caused by stenosis will be more pronounced with less diameter reduction in a _low_ resistance system.

20. Under normal conditions with exercise, blood flow _increases_ by at least three to five times the resting value.

Short Answer

1. How is Bernoulli's principle applied to the circulatory system?

   It's used Cardiac imaging. By measuring the velocity at stenotic valve, one can determine the pressure drop across a valve and thus the clinical significance

2. In the human circulatory system, when do viscous and inertial losses occur?

> It occures whenever blood is forced to change direction or velocity

3. Why does the velocity of the blood decrease as the blood travels from the aorta to the arterioles?

> because the change in size of the vessels

4. According to Poiseuille's Law, how is volume flow impacted by changes in vessel radius?

> If the radius of a vessel changes, it will have a significant impact on flow because it is the radius to the forth power, which is directly proportional to flow

5. Why is hydraulic filtering necessary in the circulatory system?

> Hydraulic filtering converts the intermittent output of the heart to a steady flow through the capillaries, which ensures adequate exchange of nutrients and wastes

6. How does capacitance in the arterial system change with age?

> Capacitance decreases with age the vessel wall becomes stiffer with age

7. What are the main factors that control peripheral circulation?

> Centrally by the nervous system and locally by conditions at the tissue bed

8. How does a critical stenosis affect pressure and flow?

> a critical stenosis varies with the resistance of the run-off bed

IMAGE EVALUATION/PATHOLOGY

Review the images and answer the following questions.

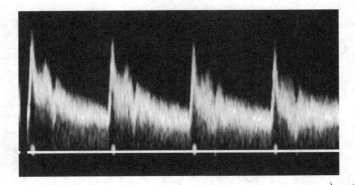

1. From this Doppler spectrum:
   1. What type of distal vascular bed does this vessel feed? ~~heart~~ *low resistance* regions with constant high metabolic demand
   2. Why does this type of vascular bed result in this waveform? the arterioles are open to allow a great deal of oxygen an nutrients
   3. Give an example of a vessel that would demonstrate this type of waveform. ICA

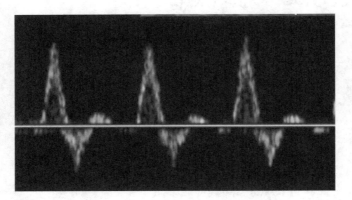

2. From this Doppler spectrum:
   1. What type of distal vascular bed does this vessel feed? ~~eca~~ high resistance
   2. Why does this type of vascular bed result in this waveform? eca subclavian
   3. Give an example of a vessel that would demonstrate this type of waveform. ECA

CASE STUDY

1. A patient presents to the vascular lab for duplex ultrasound evaluation of the carotid artery system. During the evaluation, the vascular technologist notices turbulence in the proximal common carotid artery. Discuss the factors that contribute to turbulence and indicate the circumstances that may have led to turbulent flow being noted in this artery.

2. A patient presents to the vascular lab for evaluation of peripheral arterial occlusive disease. During the evaluation, blood pressures are taken at the patient's ankles both before and after exercise. Before exercise, the patient's ankle pressures are noted to be within a normal range; however, after exercise, the ankle pressures are noted to be significantly lower. Why might this change occur?

blood pressure distal to an arterial lesion will be decreased with mild to moderate disease. Exercise will further decrease in peripheral pressure

Venous Physiology

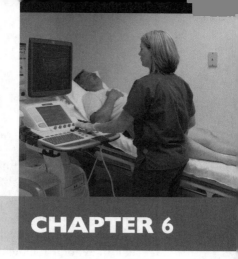

REVIEW OF GLOSSARY TERMS

Matching

Match the key terms with their definitions.

KEY TERMS

1. _____ hydrostatic pressure

2. _____ transmural pressure

3. _____ edema

4. _____ venous valvular insufficiency

DEFINITION

a. The pressure exerted on the walls of a vessel
b. Excessive accumulation of fluid in cells, tissues, or cavities of the body
c. The pressure within the vascular system because of the weight of a column of blood
d. Abnormal retrograde flow in veins

CHAPTER REVIEW

Multiple Choice

Complete each question by circling the best answer.

1. Approximately how much blood does the venous portion of the vascular system hold?
   a. 66% to 67% of the total volume of blood
   b. One-third of the total volume of blood
   c. 3% to 4% of the total volume of blood
   d. Half of the total volume of blood

2. Which statement about the resistance of the venous system is NOT correct?
   a. Veins offer resistance to flow through increase in pressure.
   b. Veins offer natural resistance to flow in some areas of the body.
   c. An elliptical shape in the vein increases the resistance.
   d. A circular shape in the vein decreases the resistance.

3. Which veins do NOT offer natural resistance to flow in the venous system?
   a. the subclavian veins
   b. the femoral veins
   c. the jugular veins
   d. the inferior vena cava

4. In a 6-foot-tall individual in a standing position, hydrostatic pressure will add approximately how much to the measured pressure at the ankle?
   a. 170 mm Hg
   b. 100 mm Hg
   c. 15 mm Hg
   d. 20 mm Hg

5. What is the minimum pressure inside a vein needed to prevent it from collapsing?
   a. −50 mm Hg
   b. −5 mm Hg
   c. 5 mm Hg
   d. −35 mm Hg

6. What is the pressure gradient across the capillary bed in an uplifted arm owing to the change in hydrostatic pressure?
   a. 100 mm Hg
   b. 80 mm Hg
   c. 40 mm Hg
   d. 20 mm Hg

7. Once a vein has acquired a circular shape, how can the volume of blood in the vessel only change with?
   a. large increase of pressure
   b. little increase of pressure
   c. no increase of pressure
   d. negative pressure

8. When an individual moves from a supine to a standing position, which of the following pressures specific to the venous system increases?
   a. osmotic pressure
   b. hydrostatic pressure
   c. transmural pressure
   d. gravitational force

9. Which of the following is NOT a force influencing the movement of fluid at the level of the capillaries (in or out of the surrounding tissue)?
   a. intracapillary pressure
   b. interstitial osmotic pressure
   c. capillary osmotic pressure
   d. transmural pressure

10. How does the action of the calf muscle pump, under normal circumstances, offset fluid loss in interstitial tissue?
    a. It helps increase the venous pressure.
    b. It helps decrease the venous pressure.
    c. It helps decrease the osmotic pressure.
    d. It helps decrease the interstitial pressure.

11. Under normal circumstances, the inspiration phase of respiration results in all of the following EXCEPT:
    a. an ascent of the diaphragm.
    b. a descent of the diaphragm.
    c. an increase in intra-abdominal pressure.
    d. a decrease in intrathoracic pressure.

12. With total or partial thrombosis of proximal major veins of the lower extremities, what action is not unusual for the flow profile from distal nonoccluded veins to do?
    a. To change from continuous to phasic
    b. To change from phasic to pulsatile
    c. To change from pulsatile to phasic
    d. To change from phasic to continuous

13. Which of the following is essential to ensure the proper functioning of the calf muscle pump under normal conditions?
    a. properly functioning valves
    b. well-developed gastrocnemius muscle venous sinusoids
    c. well-developed soleal muscle venous sinusoids
    d. a superficial venous system

14. How much pressure can be generated by the contraction of an efficient calf muscle pump under normal conditions?
    a. At least 50 mm Hg
    b. At least 15 mm Hg
    c. At least 200 mm Hg
    d. At least 5 mm Hg

15. How are primary varicose veins distinguished from secondary varicose veins?
    a. Do not affect the small saphenous vein.
    b. Develop in the absence of deep venous thrombosis.
    c. Do not rely on the calf muscle pump.
    d. Do not rely on proper valve closure in the deep veins.

16. Increased pressure in the distal venous system seen in secondary varicose veins is because of all of the following EXCEPT:
    a. distal obstruction of the venous system.
    b. bidirectional flow in the perforators.
    c. increased pressure in the deep venous system.
    d. increased pressure in the superficial venous system.

17. What is a fibrin cuff?
    a. By product of the breakdown of a thrombus.
    b. Fibrin accumulation around the capillaries.
    c. The trapping of fibrin and white blood cells in the venules.
    d. The movement of fibrin and other plasma proteins into the tissue.

18. What caused venous distension during pregnancy?
    a. an increased venous flow velocity
    b. incompetent valves
    c. an increased compliance of the veins
    d. compression of the superior vena cava

19. What does a continuous venous flow profile from veins of the lower extremities mean?
    a. The flow is no longer responsive to pressure changes from respiration.
    b. The flow is increased in pregnancy.
    c. It is the result of incompetent valves in the deep system.
    d. It is the result of incompetent valves in the superficial system.

20. What are the major physiology components governing blood flow in the venous system?
    a. venous capacitance
    b. transmural pressure
    c. hydrostatic pressure
    d. all of the above

Fill-in-the-Blank

1. Veins are known as the capacitance vessels of the body because they act as a _____.

2. The cross-sectional area of a distended vein could be _____ larger than the area of the corresponding artery.

3. The fact that veins are usually paired in many area of the body increases the _____ of the vascular system.

4. A major force affecting the venous system is _____.

5. Hydrostatic pressure is measured by the density of the blood × the acceleration due to gravity × _____.

6. The hydrostatic pressure in an arm raised straight above the head would be _____.

7. Transmural pressure is equal to the _____ between the intravascular pressure in the vein and the pressure in the surrounding tissue.

8. When standing, low-pressure compression stockings have a(n) _____ effect in reducing the venous pressure and volume.

9. Fluid, which normally moves to the interstitial space of tissue, is usually absorbed by _____ vessels.

10. The pressure exerted by a fluid when there is a difference in the concentrations of solutes across a semipermeable membrane is _____ pressure.

11. The _____ plays an important role in the regulation of venous return to the heart by changing the intra-thoracic and intra-abdominal pressures.

12. In venous thrombosis, the influence of respiration and changing intra-abdominal pressure has _____ effect on the pressure gradient from the legs.

13. The calf muscle pump assists in the return of venous flow to the heart when an individual is standing because it works against _____ pressure.

14. Venous reflux in the distal calf during the contraction of the calf muscles under normal conditions is prevented by valve closure in _____.

15. Primary varicose veins rarely involve the _____ vein.

16. In secondary varicose veins, the flow in the perforators can be _____, which increases the pressure within the superficial system.

17. A serious consequence of venous insufficiency and secondary varicose veins is venous stasis _____.

18. During pregnancy, increased venous compliance, pressure, and distension coupled with decreased velocity of venous flow out of the legs can contribute to the development of _____.

19. Typically, varicose veins become _____ with subsequent pregnancies.

20. The venous Doppler signals observed during an ultrasound examination are a direct result of venous _____.

Short Answer

1. How do veins vary their resistance to blood flow?

2. When standing, what does increased hydrostatic pressure in both the arteries and the veins ensure?

3. What determines the shape of a vein? What shapes do veins take based on this quantity?

4. What actions occur during inspiration and expiration that impact venous blood flow?

5. What role do the calf muscle pump and perforators play in primary varicose veins?

6. What are the underlying issues related to venous blood flow that help to create venous stasis ulcers?

CASE STUDY

1. A patient presents to the vascular lab for evaluation of the lower extremity venous system. During the examination, the technologist notices a continuous venous flow pattern in the common femoral vein. What do these results suggest?

2. A 45-year-old female patient presents to the vascular lab with visible varicose veins. Upon questioning, the patient states that she had deep vein thrombosis previously during pregnancy. Based on this history, would you expect primary or secondary varicose veins and which venous systems might be affected by venous valvular insufficiency?

PART THREE

CEREBROVASCULAR

The Extracranial Duplex Ultrasound Examination

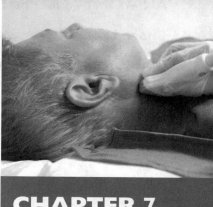

CHAPTER 7

REVIEW OF GLOSSARY TERMS

Matching

Match the key terms with their definitions.

KEY TERMS

1. __C__ transient ischemic attack
2. __d__ carotid bulb
3. __f__ bruit
4. __e__ spectral analysis
5. __b__ spectral broadening
6. __a__ Doppler angle

DEFINITION

a. Most commonly defined as the angle between the line of the Doppler ultrasound beam and the arterial wall (also referred to as the "angle of insonation"). This is a key variable in the Doppler equation used to calculate flow velocity

b. An increase in the "width" of the spectral waveform (frequency band) or "filling-in" of the normal clear area under the systolic peak. This represents turbulent blood flow associated with arterial lesions

c. An episode of stroke-like neurologic symptoms that typically lasts for a few minutes to several hours and then resolves completely. This is caused by temporary interruption of the blood supply to the brain in the distribution of a cerebral artery

d. A slight dilation involving variable portions of the distal common and proximal internal carotid arteries, often including the origin of the external carotid artery. This is where the baroreceptors assisting in reflex blood pressure control are located. The carotid bulb tends to be most prominent in normal young individuals

e. Signal processing technique that displays the complete frequency and amplitude content of the Doppler flow signal. The spectral information is usually presented as waveforms with frequency (converted to a velocity scale) on the vertical axis, time on the horizontal axis, and amplitude indicated by a grayscale

f. An abnormal "blowing" or "swishing" sound heard with a stethoscope while auscultating over an artery, such as the carotid. The sound results from vibrations that are transmitted through the tissues when blood flows through a stenotic artery.

ANATOMY AND PHYSIOLOGY REVIEW

Image Labeling

Complete the labels in the images that follow.

ICA Distal

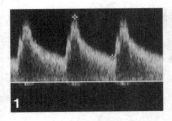

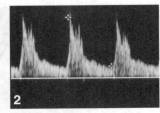

ICA Prox

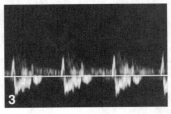

bulb, flowseperation

1. If the above Doppler waveforms were from a normal (nondiseased) internal carotid artery, label what the wave-forms would best represent.

CCA

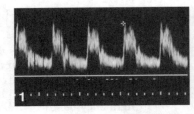

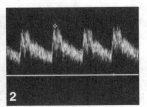

ICA

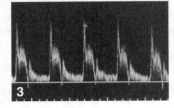

ECA

2. If the following Doppler waveforms were taken from normal (nondiseased) vessels, label the artery that best characterizes the flow based on the waveforms' contours.

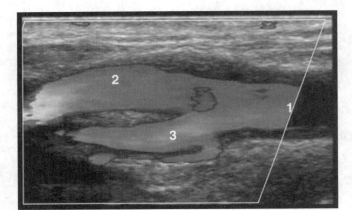

CCA
ICA
ECA

3. Assuming normal anatomy, label the vessels.

CHAPTER REVIEW

Multiple Choice

Complete each question by circling the best answer.

1. What is the secondary goal of examination of the extracranial carotid artery system by duplex ultrasound?
   a. To identify patients at risk for stroke
   b. To diagnose fibromuscular dysplasia
   c. To document progression of disease
   d. To screen for iatrogenic problems

2. Which transducer is most commonly used to perform a duplex evaluation of the extracranial cerebrovascular system?
   a. 7-4 MHz linear array
   b. 8-5 MHz curvilinear array
   c. 4-1 MHz phased array
   d. 5-3 MHz phased array

3. A patient presents to the vascular lab for a carotid-vertebral duplex examination. Upon questioning, the patient reveals a 2-week history of intermittent blindness in the right eye. The symptoms resolve within a few seconds. What would these symptoms indicate?
   a. CVA
   b. RIND
   c. TIA
   d. DVT

4. How should the patient's head be positioned in order to expedite a carotid-vertebral duplex examination?
   a. Head straight forward and elevated on a pillow.
   b. Head rotated 45 degrees away from side being examined with a pillow under shoulders.
   c. Head rotated 90 degrees toward side being examined supported by a pillow.
   d. Head straight with a rolled-up towel placed under the neck.

5. What is the most common technique used to identify the vertebral artery?
   a. View the common carotid artery and angle the transducer slightly posteriorly.
   b. View the subclavian artery and angle the transducer superiorly.
   c. View the basilar artery and angle the transducer inferiorly.
   d. View the vertebral processes and angle the transducer medially.

6. When qualifying the appearance of plaque by ultrasound, the use of which of the following terms is discouraged owing to poor reliability?
   a. homogeneous/heterogeneous
   b. smooth/irregular
   c. ulcerated
   d. calcified

7. As plaque develops and fills the carotid bulb, what change can be expected in the Doppler waveform at this level?
   a. extremely high velocities
   b. disappearance of normal flow separation
   c. helical flow around the plaque
   d. development of "steal" waveform

8. Which of the following will NOT result in symmetrical (i.e., seen in both carotid and sometimes vertebral arterial systems) changes in the Doppler spectra?
   a. aortic valve or root stenosis
   b. brain death
   c. subclavian steal
   d. intra-aortic balloon pump

9. In a normally hemodynamically low-resistance system or vessel, such as the internal carotid and vertebral arteries, what will a change to high-resistance pattern suggest?
   a. proximal stenosis or occlusion
   b. distal stenosis or occlusion
   c. steal syndrome
   d. normal change because of exercise

10. What is reactive hyperemia, a provocative maneuver used during the duplex evaluation of the extracranial cerebrovascular system, used to demonstrate?
    a. The diagnosis of brain death.
    b. A change from latent or partial to complete subclavian steal.
    c. The existence of a unilateral congenital small vertebral artery.
    d. The effect of an intra-aortic balloon pump.

11. Which of the following is NOT "sound" advice for sonographers who wish to prevent repetitive stress injuries while scanning?
    a. Be ambidextrous.
    b. Arrange bed and equipment to be close to patient.
    c. Remain well hydrated during the day.
    d. Avoid doing stretching exercises.

12. Which of the following is NOT a characteristic of normal Doppler waveform contour?
    a. brisk systolic acceleration
    b. sharp systolic peak
    c. increased spectral broadening
    d. clear spectral window

13. Why do Doppler waveforms in the common carotid arteries display a contour suggestive of relatively low-resistance flow?
    a. 70% of its flow supplies the ICA
    b. 90% of its flow supplies the ICA
    c. 70% of its flow supplies the ECA
    d. 90% of its flow supplies the ECA

14. What type of flow is characterized by a blunted, resistive waveform that often occurs before total occlusion?
    a. steal flow
    b. tardus parvus flow
    c. bidirectional flow
    d. string sign flow

15. Which statement on power Doppler is FALSE?
    a. It represents the amplitude of the Doppler signal instead of frequency shift.
    b. It depends on the angle of insonation.
    c. It does not give information about flow direction.
    d. It can detect low-flow states.

16. A patient presents to the vascular lab with a severe distal CCA obstruction; however, the internal carotid and external carotid artery remain patent. What is this lesion typically called?
    a. subclavian steal syndrome
    b. string sign lesion
    c. choke lesion
    d. tardus parvus lesion

17. During duplex evaluation of the internal carotid artery, peak systolic velocities are noted to 532 cm/s and end diastolic velocities are 167 cm/s. According to the University of Washington criteria, into what stenosis category would these findings fall?
    a. 16% to 49% stenosis
    b. 50% to 79% stenosis
    c. 80% to 99% stenosis
    d. occlusion

18. For subclavian steal syndrome or phenomenon to occur, where does a severe stenosis or an occlusion need to be present?
    a. The subclavian artery distal to the vertebral artery origin.
    b. The left subclavian artery or brachiocephalic artery proximal to the vertebral artery origin.
    c. The origin of the common carotid arteries.
    d. Anywhere in the brachial arteries.

19. Which of the following would affect pulsed Doppler spectrum contour in all vessels of the extracranial cerebrovascular arterial system even when no disease is present?
    a. low-cardiac output
    b. aortic root stenosis
    c. intra-aortic balloon pump
    d. All of the above

20. During duplex evaluation of the carotid artery system, velocities in the external carotid artery reached 250 cm/s, and turbulence was noted just after the area of increased velocity. What do these findings suggest?
    a. >50% stenosis
    b. Normal findings for the ECA
    c. 50% to 79% stenosis
    d. >80% stenosis

Fill-in-the-Blank

1. The primary goal of an examination of the extracranial cerebrovascular system by duplex ultrasound is to identify patients at risk for _Stroke_.

2. Approximately _1/3_ of neck bruits are related to significant stenosis of the internal carotid artery.

3. Lesions or stenoses in the internal carotid arteries can be present without _neurologic_ symptoms.

4. High-grade stenoses of the internal carotid arteries, as flow restricting lesions, are rarely the primary cause of neurologic symptoms because of _collateral flow_

5. Flow separation can be seen in the carotid bulb and will be represented by brief flow *reversal*.

6. Transient symptoms manifested as a difficulty to speak are termed as *dysphasia*.

7. Neurologic deficits lasting between 24 and 72 hours are classified as *RIND*.

8. If significant flow turbulence is noted in the proximal right common carotid, it becomes imperative to examine the *Brachiocephalic artery*.

9. There are usually two recommended methods to distinguish the internal from the external carotid artery. In one method, one would perform *temporal tap* to demonstrate oscillations on the Doppler spectrum.

10. The use of a curved or phased array transducer is recommended for the examination of the distal internal carotid arteries, particularly in patients with tortuous vessels, fibromuscular dysplasia, or vessels that are *deeper* than usual.

11. In order to evaluate the subclavian artery, the transducer is placed in a(n) *transverse* orientation at the base of the neck.

12. The internal features of plaque found in the extracranial cerebrovascular system are usually related to the *echogenicity* of the plaque.

13. Bleeding within a plaque underneath the fibrous cap (intraplaque hemorrhage) can cause the plaque to become *unstable*.

14. Dissection of the intima, particularly in common carotid arteries, could be confused with artifacts from the wall of *IJV*.

15. *iatrogenic* injury is defined as any adverse patient condition that is induced inadvertently by a health care provider during a diagnostic procedure or intervention.

16. "Latent," "hesitant," "alternating," and "complete" are terms usually describing the stages of *Steel phenomenon*.

17. The waveform contour distal to a significant stenosis is often referred to as a *tardus parvus* pattern, characterized by damped, rounded waveform with decreased velocity and delayed acceleration.

18. In the presence of significant common carotid stenosis, the ICA/CCA ratio criteria are *not valid*.

19. *Power* Doppler is particularly helpful in detecting extremely low-flow velocities, including string sign flow.

20. According to the criteria developed by the University of Washington, the stenosis categories below the 50% threshold are differentiated from one another by the presence or absence of flow separation, the extent of spectral *broadening*, and the amount of plaque visualized.

Short Answer

1. How can the internal and external carotid arteries be safely differentiated?

The ECA is typically located medial to the ICA and has multiple branches and a temporal tap can be used which shows oscillations down the ECA that can be seen

2. What is the primary criterion for determining an internal carotid artery stenosis? Once this primary threshold has been exceeded, what is the secondary criterion used to further categorize disease?

the PSV. PSV > 125 cm/s is consistent with a > 50% stenosis. The EDV > 140 cm/s indicates a > 80% stenosis

3. According to the Consensus Panel recommendations, what findings are consistent with occlusion of the internal carotid artery?

No detectable patent lumen on grayscale imaging and no flow with PW Doppler, color Doppler, or power Doppler

4. What did NASCET determine to be the best criteria for determining a >70% stenosis?

> 70% stenosis as PSV > 230 cm/s or an ICA to CCA PSV ratio of 4.0 or greater

5. How is stenosis determined in extracranial vessels other than the internal carotid artery?

a focal velocity increase in PSV twice that of a normal proximal site (velocity > 2)

IMAGE EVALUATION/PATHOLOGY

Review the images and answer the following questions.

pg 80

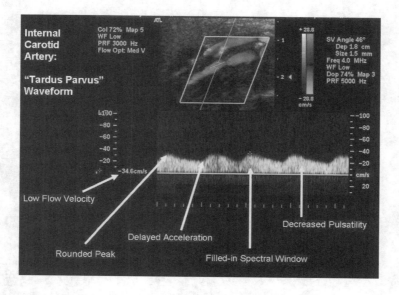

1. Based on the characteristics of the Doppler spectrum from this internal carotid artery, what is a possible cause of this waveform contour?

    it's distal to a significant stenosis

    proximal stenosis

pg. 80

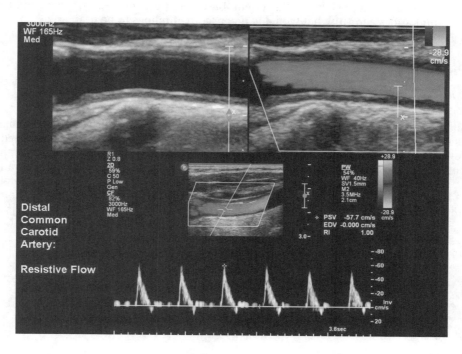

2. Based on the Doppler characteristics seen in this common carotid artery, what is a possible cause of this waveform contour?

    ipsilateral ICA occlusion

    Distal occlusion

CASE STUDY

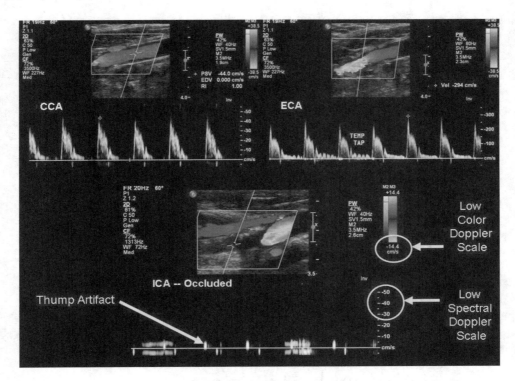

1. A 72-year-old female patient presents to the vascular lab for carotid artery duplex evaluation. Upon examination, these images were obtained from the left carotid system. Based on these images, (a) what can be concluded about the left internal carotid artery and (b) what would you expect the findings to be in the right carotid system (assuming no significant stenosis)?

   A.) The left ICA is completely occluded shown by lack of flow and higher than normal resistance waveform in the CCA

   B. The right velocities and waveforms would likely fall within normal parameters; however they could be elevated because of compensatory flow

2. A 68-year-old male patient presents to the vascular lab for carotid-vertebral artery duplex examination. Brachial blood pressures in this patient are noted to be 142 mm Hg on the right and 114 mm Hg on the left. During the duplex examination, the bilateral carotid artery systems are noted to be free of significant stenosis; however, increased velocities are noted in the left subclavian artery. Additionally, an alternating flow type waveform is noted in the left vertebral artery, whereas the right vertebral artery demonstrates normal Doppler waveform contour. Based on these findings, (a) what disease process is occurring in this patient and (b) what additional test could be performed to help augment these findings?

   a) Latent subclavian steal is occurring, based on left subclavian stenosis

   b) Reactive hyperemia could be performed to show the change from latent steal to complete steal

Uncommon Pathology of the Carotid System

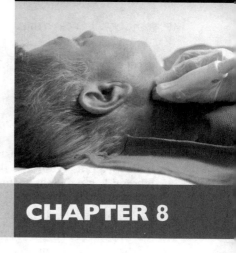

CHAPTER 8

REVIEW OF GLOSSARY TERMS

Matching

Match the key terms with their definitions.

KEY TERMS

1. __C__ aneurysm

2. __h__ arteritis

3. __d__ carotid body tumor

4. __b__ dissection

5. __g__ fibromuscular dysplasia

6. __e__ intimal flap

7. __a__ pseudoaneurysm

8. __f__ tortuosity

DEFINITION

a. A dilation of an artery with disruption of one or more layers of the vessel wall causing an expanding hematoma; also called false aneurysm

b. A tear along the inner layer of an artery that results in the splitting or separation of the walls of a blood vessel

c. A localized dilatation of the wall of an artery

d. A benign mass (also called paraganglioma or chemo-dectoma) of the carotid body, which is a small round mass at the carotid bifurcation

e. A small tear in the wall of a blood vessel, resulting in a portion of the intima and part of the media pro-truding into the lumen of the vessel; this free portion of the blood vessel wall may appear to move with pulsations in flow

f. The quality of being tortuous, winding, and twisting

g. Abnormal growth and development of the muscular layer of an artery wall with fibrosis and collagen de-position causing stenosis

h. Inflammation of an artery

CHAPTER REVIEW

Multiple Choice

Complete each question by circling the best answer.

1. A pulsatile mass at the base of the neck may be indicative (and often mistaken) for an aneurysm, when it is most likely tortuosity of which of the following?
   a. the proximal subclavian artery
   b. the proximal vertebral artery
   c. the proximal common carotid
   d. the proximal internal jugular vein

2. Which of the following is NOT a characteristic of the flow in a secondary lumen created by a tear or dissection?
   a. same direction of flow as in the true lumen
   b. reverse direction of flow, exiting the false lumen through a secondary proximal tear
   c. an alternate antegrade/retrograde flow pattern in and out of the false lumen
   d. high velocities as would be seen in stenosis

3. What is a likely source of the symptoms in patients under 50 years of age presenting to the vascular lab with symptoms of stroke (without typical risk factors)?
   a. dissection of one of the carotid vessels
   b. stenosis due to atherosclerosis
   c. carotid body tumor
   d. tortuous distal ICA with kinking of the vessel

4. When performing Doppler on a tortuous internal carotid artery, how should the cursor be aligned if a velocity measurement must be made on a curved segment of the artery?
   a. Set the angle cursor so that it is at the inside of the curve.
   b. Set the angle cursor so the middle of the cursor is parallel to the walls and center stream.
   c. Set the angle cursor so the end of the cursor is parallel to the walls and at the highest point of the curve
   d. Set the angle cursor where the highest velocities are indicated by color Doppler.

5. Which of the following is a major feature that should be present for a diagnosis of dissection?
   a. a color pattern clearly showing two flow directions in the true lumen
   b. identifiable thrombus within false lumen
   c. atherosclerosis along the posterior wall
   d. a hyperechoic (white/bright) line in the lumen of the artery

6. Which condition consists of a repetitive pattern of narrowing and small dilatation in an internal carotid artery, giving the appearance of a "string of beads"?
   a. dissection
   b. aneurysms
   c. fibromuscular dysplasia
   d. presence of enlarged lymph nodes

7. In a patient with hypertension, incidental diagnosis of fibromuscular dysplasia in the carotid artery system should lead to follow-up evaluation of which vessel(s)?
   a. subclavian arteries
   b. renal arteries
   c. intracranial vessels
   d. aorta

8. Which of the following describes a vessel diameter measuring >200% of the diameter of a normal section of the ICA or >150% of the CCA?
   a. true aneurysm of carotid vessels
   b. large carotid bulb
   c. normal carotid bulb
   d. pseudoaneurysm

9. What is the distinguishing flow pattern in the neck of a pseudoaneurysm?
   a. low-resistance arterial pattern
   b. alternating, to-and-fro pattern
   c. phasic venous pattern
   d. high-velocity stenotic pattern

10. Why is it important to thoroughly evaluate the vessel wall of the artery where a perforation led to a pseudoaneurysm?
    a. Aliasing is very likely at the area of the perforation.
    b. Dissection may occur along the vessel wall.
    c. Thrombosis is likely to occur in that area.
    d. Plaque is often present in that area.

11. When is radiation-induced arterial injury suspected?
    a. The plaque is widespread.
    b. The plaque has high echogenicity.
    c. The plaque is vascularized.
    d. The "plaque" is isolated and located in an atypical area.

12. What are the major forms of arteritis found in the carotid system?
    a. Takayasu's disease and temporal arteritis *(circled)*
    b. giant cell arteritis and FMD
    c. FMD and CBT
    d. none of the above

13. A 62-year-old female presents to the vascular lab a pulsatile mass in her neck, and hoarseness in her voice is noticed. What would you suspect?
    a. carotid body tumor *(circled)*
    b. spontaneous dissection
    c. fibromuscular dysplasia
    d. common carotid artery aneurysm *(circled)*

14. Why is it crucial to survey the entire visible length of the vessel when evaluating the superficial temporal artery for signs of temporal arteritis?
    a. The inflamed area is not continuous. *(circled)*
    b. The vessel is often tortuous.
    c. Dissections are often present locally. *(circled)*
    d. Areas of dilatation are present locally.

15. A 30-year-old female presents to the vascular lab with decreased radial pulses and upper extremities claudication. What would you suspect?
    a. Takayasu's disease *(circled)*
    b. giant cell arteritis
    c. carotid body tumor
    d. spontaneous dissection

16. A 60-year-old female presents to the vascular lab with history of headaches and tenderness in the temporal area as well as jaw claudication. What would you suspect?
    a. Takayasu's disease
    b. carotid body tumor
    c. giant cell arteritis *(circled)*
    d. spontaneous dissection

17. A 25-year-old male involved in competitive bicycle racing presents in the vascular lab with symptoms of headaches and subtle neurologic changes after a crash on the race course. What would you suspect?
    a. giant cell arteritis
    b. spontaneous dissection *(circled)*
    c. Takayasu's disease
    d. carotid body tumor

18. A 75-year-old male with long-lasting history of COPD presents in the vascular lab for evaluation of his carotid arteries. An incidental mass is visualized at the carotid bifurcation on the right side, splaying the internal and external carotid arteries. What would you suspect?
    a. spontaneous dissection
    b. carotid body tumor *(circled)*
    c. giant cell arteritis
    d. Takayasu's disease

19. You are asked to evaluate a pulsatile neck mass in an 80-year-old female with recent placement of a central line in the right internal jugular vein. What would you suspect?
    a. a pseudoaneurysm *(circled)*
    b. an enlarged lymph node
    c. a carotid body tumor
    d. a dissection

20. A 50-year-male with history of non-Hodgkin lymphoma treated with radiation presents in the vascular lab with some neurologic changes. What would you suspect?
    a. carotid body tumor
    b. enlarged lymph nodes
    c. radiation-induced arterial disease *(circled)*
    d. dissection

Fill-in-the-Blank

1. Application of flow-velocity criteria for the accurate evaluation of a tortuous internal carotid artery is difficult. It is therefore recommended that a combination of ___Color___ imaging together with Doppler velocities will demonstrate the suspected area.

2. A dissection of an arterial wall may create what is commonly referred to as a ___false___ lumen.

3. It is important to obtain a thorough medical or lifestyle history to evaluate for subtle trauma to the neck in patients presenting with ___Spontaneous dissection___

4. With dissections that appear to be spontaneous, the primary risk fact is often ___hypertension___

5. Fibromuscular dysplasia affects predominantly _renal_ arteries.

6. One of the best "tools" available on duplex ultrasound to clearly depict the "string of beads" appearance associated with fibromuscular dysplasia in the internal carotid artery is _power Doppler_

7. The Doppler spectrum in the arteries found within a carotid body tumor will typically display _low_ -resistance characteristic.

8. To avoid overestimating the diameter of a carotid artery aneurysm, measurements should be taken at the widest diameter in a _longitudinal_ view along the axis of flow.

9. Penetrating trauma to the neck, presence of a bypass graft in the carotid system, or history of endarterectomy may (although rare) lead to the formation of _pseudoaneurysm_ .

10. The area of highest narrowing seen with radiation-induced arterial injury tends to be at the _distal_ end of the stenotic area.

11. A long, homogeneous narrowing typically seen in the subclavian artery of a young female patient would suggest _Takayasu syndrome_

12. In a transverse view, a "halo" surrounding the outer layer of the facial artery may suggest _Temporal arteritis_

13. Two clearly different Doppler spectra seen as Doppler sampling on each side of a "white" line in an arterial lumen suggests _dissection_ .

14. The typical color-flow pattern within a pseudoaneurysm in a transverse view will demonstrate a(n) _yin-yang_ appearance, with red on half of the mass and blue on the other.

15. Inflammation of an artery, which may result in the breakdown of the structure of the arterial wall, is generally termed as _Arteritis_ .

16. Injury to the vasa vasorum, located in the media of the arterial wall and resulting in fibrosis of the portion of the wall, is the basis for lesions seen with _RIAI_ .

17. Typically, nonmalignant paragangliomas of the neck are also called _Carotid Body Tumor_ .

18. An abnormal growth of smooth muscle cells in the media of the internal carotid artery has been shown to be the underlying pathologic mechanism of _Fibromuscular Dysplasia_

19. It is believed that possibly one-fourth of the adult population present with some degree of _tortuosity_ bilaterally, predominantly in the distal internal carotid arteries.

20. To ensure that velocity changes (particularly sudden increases) in a tortuous vessel are the result of a stenosis rather than sudden changes in direction of flow, one should thoroughly examined the vessels in _B-mode_ .

Short Answer

1. How can a pseudoaneurysm be differentiated from an enlarged lymph node?

pseudo aneurysms have a neck that connects to the vessel and has a to-and-fro flow pattern
lymph nodes have low-resistance arterial pattern & venous flow

2. In addition to ultrasound findings, what should the vascular technologist pay attention to when assessing a patient suspected of an uncommon vascular pathology?

the patients history

IMAGE EVALUATION/PATHOLOGY

Review the images and answer the following questions.

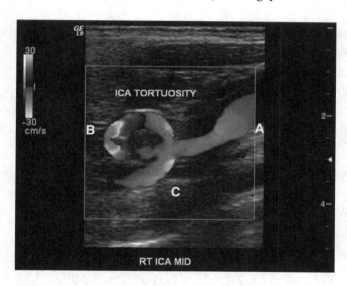

1. Describe the flow direction in areas A, B, and C (in relation to the transducer).

A - Away
B - toward
C - away

2. In area B, how would you label the mosaic of color seen?

Aliasing

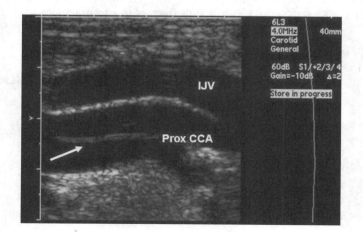

3. What is the arrow most likely pointing to?

Dissection
false lumen

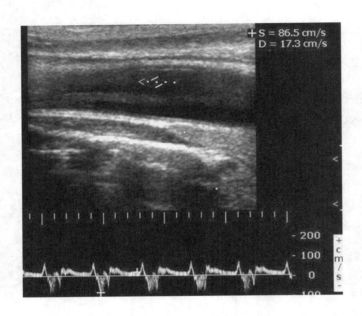

4. What would the Doppler spectrum seen here (in the context of the pathology depicted) suggest regarding the sample volume?

pseudo aneurysms have a

False lumen

CASE STUDY

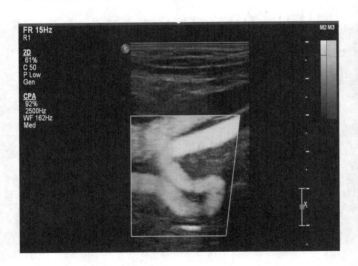

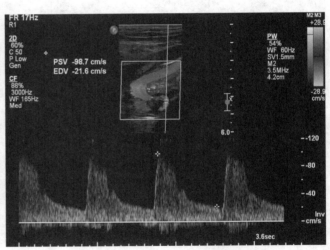

1. These two images were taken at the same level in a patient. Which artery is most likely depicted in these images? Why? Which techniques are used in each image to show flow? What is the advantage of using each technique? The flow velocities were recorded as: PSV: 98.7 cm/s and EDV: 21.6 cm/s. What is missing? Discuss the accuracy of the data.

power Doppler on the ICA   pulse wave + color Doppler

there is no angle on the Doppler cursor

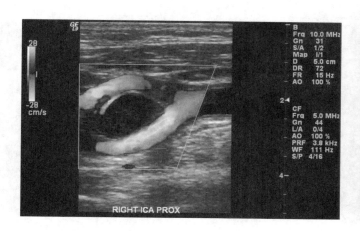

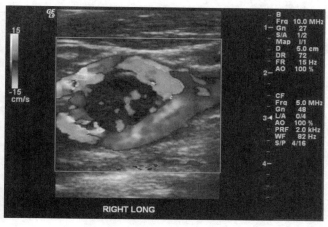

2. These images were taken at the level of the bifurcation of internal and external carotid arteries. What rather uncommon pathology is most likely represented in this image? Describe the relevant points leading to your conclusion. Between image 1 and image 2, the sonographer changed one of the settings for color display. Explain the rationale for the choice. What alternate tool could have been used? What symptoms might this patient have?

Carotid body tumor

The color Doppler was lowered to show the CBT is highly vascular

Symtoms of CBT are discomfort in the area, dysphagia, headaches, a change in voice

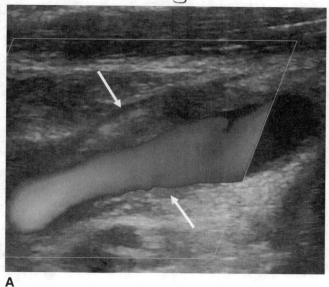

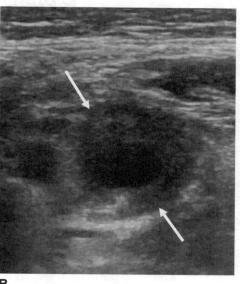

A   B

3. A 69-year-old female presented to the vascular lab with jaw claudication, visual disturbances, and tenderness over her temple. This image was taken during the ultrasound examination. What is suggested by this image? What other vessels may be impacted?

Temporal arteritis
Superficial temporal artery
aortic arch & carotid vessels, ECA & its branches

Ultrasound Following Surgery and Intervention

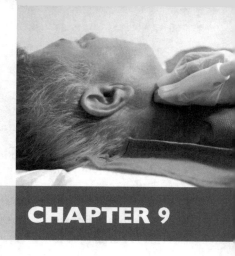

REVIEW OF GLOSSARY TERMS

Matching

Match the key terms with their definitions.

KEY TERMS

1. _____ carotid artery stenting

2. _____ carotid endarterectomy

3. _____ arteriotomy

4. _____ in-stent restenosis

5. _____ polytetrafluoroethylene

DEFINITION

a. A surgical procedure during which the carotid artery is opened and plaque is removed in order to restore normal luminal diameter

b. A narrowing of the lumen of a stent, which causes a stenosis

c. A surgical incision through the wall of an artery into the lumen

d. Abbreviated PTFE, a synthetic graft material used to create grafts and blood vessel patches; a common brand name is Gore-Tex

e. A catheter-based procedure in which a metal mesh tube is deployed into an artery to keep it open, following balloon angioplasty to dilate a stenosis

CHAPTER REVIEW

Multiple Choice

Complete each question by circling the best answer.

1. Where does a typical carotid endarterectomy procedure involving a longitudinal arteriotomy begin and end?
   a. a normal distal ECA to the bulb and ICA
   b. a normal proximal CCA to ICA
   c. a normal proximal ICA to the bulb
   d. a normal distal portion of ICA into the CCA

2. Which of the following is NOT a common problem leading to stenosis at the level of the arteriotomy performed during endarterectomy?
   a. use of a patch
   b. narrowing due to sutures
   c. retained plaque
   d. hyperplastic response

3. Why does the eversion technique for carotid endarterectomy not require a patch?
   a. The sutures are at the distal taper of the ICA.
   b. The sutures are on the superficial wall of the artery.
   c. The ICA is reverted to its original position after the procedure.
   d. The sutures are at the widened area of the bulb.

4. When evaluating an endarterectomy site within 48 hours of the surgical procedure, one should be mindful of preventing infection by using all the following EXCEPT:
   a. using sterile gel.
   b. leaving the sterile dressing in place.
   c. using sterile pads.
   d. using sterile transducer cover.

5. Because of limitations in evaluating the vessels following an endarterectomy, what becomes more important to evaluate?
   a. quality of flow in the vertebral arteries
   b. quality of flow in the proximal ICA
   c. quality of flow in the distal ICA
   d. quality of flow in the contralateral ICA

6. Which malformation may be associated with neck swelling post-CEA?
   a. pseudoaneurysm
   b. hematoma
   c. infection
   d. all of the above

7. What is a perivascular fluid collection above an irregular buckling of a patch an indication of?
   a. active infection
   b. pseudoaneurysm
   c. hematoma
   d. patch rupture

8. What is stenosis at the CEA site usually considered to result from more than 24 months after an endarterectomy?
   a. neointimal hyperplasia
   b. thrombosis
   c. atherosclerotic process
   d. intimal flap

9. During duplex evaluation of a patient post-CEA, residual plaque is noted at the distal end of the surgical site, creating an abrupt edge of the arterial wall. What is this defect commonly called?
   a. intimal flap
   b. dissection
   c. shelf lesion
   d. myointimal hyperplasia

10. When might the velocity criteria established for native (nonoperated) carotid arteries NOT be valid in a post-CEA ICA?
    a. CEA with primary closure
    b. CEA with patch closure
    c. eversion CEA
    d. native criteria are not used after any CEA procedure

11. Which artery is most often used for catheter insertion for CAS?
    a. the popliteal artery
    b. the common femoral artery
    c. the brachial artery
    d. the common carotid artery

12. What is the guidewire used for CAS usually first used to deploy and position?
    a. the embolic protection device
    b. the balloon catheter
    c. the stent catheter
    d. the sheath

13. Stent distortion has been reported with mechanical forces on the neck from all the following EXCEPT:
    a. head tilting.
    b. coughing.
    c. neck rotations.
    d. swallowing.

14. For maximal efficacy, how far should a stent extend proximal and distal to the lesion?
    a. a few centimeters
    b. less than 1 mm
    c. a few millimeters
    d. more than 10 mm

15. During a duplex examination post-CAS, the stent is noted to have an irregular border with an abrupt edge. Turbulence is noted with color and spectral Doppler. What do these findings suggest?
    a. stent fracture
    b. stent deformation
    c. stent restenosis
    d. dissection

16. Which statement is true of postprocedural elevation of velocities in CAS?
    a. It is always a sign of restenosis.
    b. It is not as frequent as in CEA.
    c. It is not necessarily a sign of restenosis.
    d. It is the result of great compliance of the stent.

17. How is flow maintained to the ECA when a stent has been deployed from the CCA through the ICA?
    a. Flow is occluded to the ECA.
    b. Retrograde flow from the superficial temporal artery.
    c. Through a bypass implanted with the stent.
    d. Flow through the stent interstices.

18. During duplex assessment of a carotid artery stent, velocities at the distal end of the stent reach 350 cm/s. Turbulence is noted distal to this area. What do these findings suggest?
    a. >30% in-stent stenosis
    b. >80% in-stent stenosis
    c. >50% in-stent stenosis
    d. normal findings in a stent

19. When surveilling an ICA stent, when do the majority of >50% stenoses occur?
    a. within 18 months
    b. within 1 month
    c. within 12 months
    d. within 6 months

20. Which of the following can cause difficulties with carotid artery stents, such as restriction of balloon expansion, inadequate stent expansion, and increased risk of stent fracture?
    a. smooth, homogeneous plaque
    b. tortuous carotid artery anatomy
    c. calcified plaque
    d. intraluminal thrombus

Fill-in-the-Blank

1. True restenosis of carotid endarterectomy within the first few months after surgery is due to _____.

2. The solution most often used to reduce the potential for procedure-induced stenosis with carotid endarterectomy involves the suturing of a _____.

3. Most problems arising after a carotid endarterectomy will be located at the _____ border of the arteriotomy.

4. A vein used as surgical patch for carotid endarterectomy will often be everted such as to provide a double layer of vessel wall, with the _____ of the vein facing the lumen of the artery.

5. The eversion technique for endarterectomy involves a complete _____ of the ICA and ECA at the level of the carotid bulb.

6. It is not unusual to find entrapped air directly above the CEA site. In such case, the sonographer could image the vessels using a more _____ approach.

7. The patch and swelling associated with CEA typically lies _____ to the endarterectomy.

8. If a pseudoaneurysm is visualized after CEA, the most likely source for this pathology would be _____.

9. A potential complication with a synthetic patch is that they are more _____ than a vein patch, especially when the synthetic patch is aneurysmal.

10. The conclusion of a recent study regarding velocities of the normal ICA distal to CEA patching was that these velocities were _____ than those of nonoperated ICAs.

11. Postprocedural complications of CAS are not limited to the carotid vessels but can also be seen in the _____ artery, because it is often a path for the catheter.

12. Even though stent material is highly reflective, it does not produce _____ that may limit visualization of the stent.

13. A stent should be imaged in multiple planes, ensuring that the _____ of the stent to the surrounding plaque is complete.

14. The protrusion of the stent into the vessel lumen, together with a reduced flow channel through stent on color Doppler, indicates stent _____.

15. The single greatest concern of poststent evaluation is _____.

16. Increased manipulation of the catheter at the level of a calcified plaque may increase the _____ response and lead to restenosis.

17. When using flow-velocity criteria, the primary discriminator of significant restenosis in CAS is _____.

18. A high-grade restenosis seen in CAS should correlate with PSV of _____.

19. Dense circumferential calcification is of particular concern with CAS because it _____ balloon expansion.

20. Reintervention for either CEA or CAS would be warranted if the treated lesion leads to _____.

Short Answer

1. Why do surgeons use patch closure of the arteriotomy from carotid endarterectomy?

2. What materials are typically used for surgical patches for carotid endarterectomy?

3. Once a carotid stent has been placed and allowed to self-expand, what is the next step?

4. What sonographic imaging techniques or tools should sonographers use to evaluate stents for evidence of diffuse narrowing?

5. When would re-exploration of CEA or CAS be necessary?

IMAGE EVALUATION/PATHOLOGY

Review the images and answer the following questions.

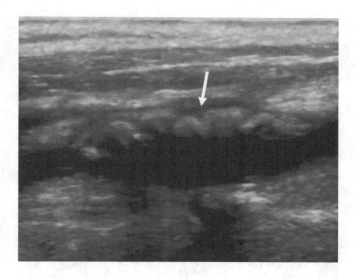

1. What is the pathology suggested in this image of a Dacron patch in a carotid artery?

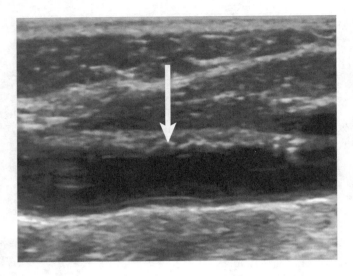

2. In this image taken on a follow-up exam following carotid endarterectomy, what is the most likely structure outlined by the arrow?

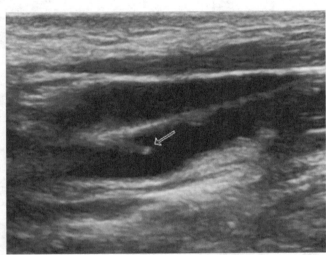

3. What does the arrow in this image most likely represent?

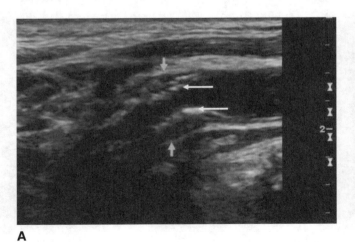

A

B

4. What is demonstrated in these images?

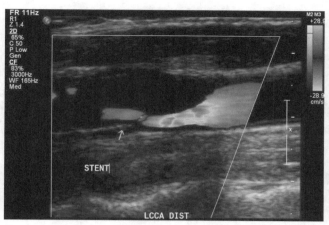

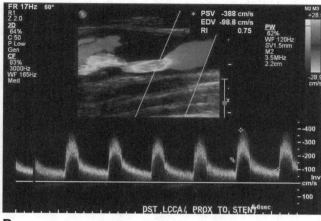

A   B

5. What is demonstrated in these images?

CASE STUDY

1. A 55-year-old male with long-standing history of type I diabetes mellitus was recently treated for a hemodynami-cally significant stenosis of his right internal carotid artery, with a stent. The procedure was done on May 2. The patient is scheduled for a follow-up ultrasound of the stented carotid a month after the procedure.

    On June 5, the patient reports to the vascular lab for a follow-up exam. The sonographer notes flow velocities in the 150 cm/s range within the stent (vs. velocities of 90 cm/s in the ICA proximal and distal to the stent). What should be considered regarding these flow velocities? What should be excluded in this first postprocedure exam?

    On December 12, the patient reports to the vascular lab for a 6-month follow-up. His physician noted a bruit dur-ing physical examination the previous day. What should be considered based on these findings? What should be recommended for follow-up based on the likely results on this exam?

2. A 78-year-old female has undergone a left carotid endarterectomy 1 month prior to presenting in your vascular lab. The procedure was done at another facility, and the notes are not available. The patient has been referred by a phy-sician based on concerns from her son that his mother seems to still experience some pain and swelling on the left side of her neck.

    Without the operative notes, what should you consider about the closure used in the procedure?

    What complications should be considered regarding this type of closure?

    When evaluating swelling from fluid accumulation from inflammation or infection, how can you distinguish swell-ing from the incision site from infection at the closure site?

Intracranial Cerebrovascular Examination

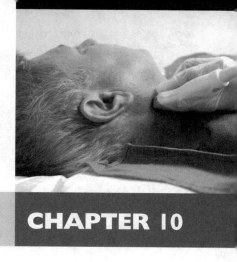

REVIEW OF GLOSSARY TERMS

Matching

Match the key terms with their definitions.

KEY TERMS

1. _____ transcranial Doppler

2. _____ transcranial duplex imaging

3. _____ circle of Willis

4. _____ vasospasm

5. _____ collateral

6. _____ pulsatility

7. _____ Lindegaard ratio

8. _____ Sviri ratio

DEFINITION

a. A noninvasive test on the intracranial cerebral blood vessels that uses ultrasound and provides both an image of the blood vessels and a graphic display of the velocities within the vessels

b. Expressed as Gosling's pulsatility index (peak systolic velocity minus end-diastolic velocity divided by the time-averaged peak velocity)

c. A vessel that parallels another vessel; a vessel that is important to maintain blood flow around another stenotic or occluded vessel

d. Middle cerebral artery (MCA) mean velocity divided by the submandibular internal carotid artery (ICA) mean velocity. This ratio is useful in differentiating increased volume flow from decreased diameter when high velocities are encountered in the MCA or intracranial ICA

e. Ratio calculation used to determine vasospasm from hyperdynamic flow in the posterior circulation. The bilateral vertebral artery velocities taken at the atlas loop are added together and averaged. This averaged velocity is then divided into the highest basilar mean velocity

f. A roughly circular anastomosis of arteries located at the base of the brain

g. A sudden constriction in a blood vessel, causing a restriction in blood flow

h. A noninvasive test that uses ultrasound to measure the velocity of blood flow through the intracranial cerebral vessels

ANATOMY AND PHYSIOLOGY REVIEW

Image Labeling

Complete the labels in the images that follow.

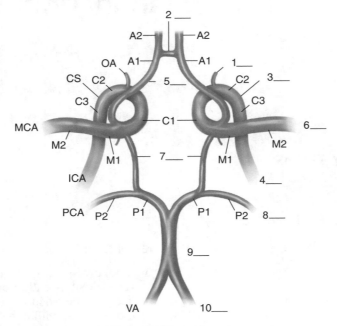

1. Circle of Willis and branches.

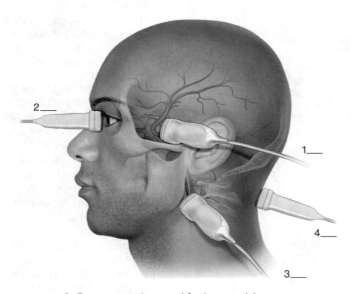

2. Four approaches used for intracranial exams.

CHAPTER REVIEW

Multiple Choice

Complete each question by circling the best answer.

1. What is the range of the average diameter of basal cerebral arteries?
   a. 1 to 3 cm
   b. 1 to 3 mm
   c. 2 to 4 cm
   d. 2 to 4 mm

2. It is estimated that 18% to 54% of individuals display variations at the level of the circle of Willis. Which of the following is NOT one of these variations?
   a. variation of number of arteries
   b. variation of caliber of vessels
   c. variation of the course of vessels
   d. variation of the origin of branches

3. Which statement about the anterior cerebral arteries is FALSE?
   a. Both arteries (right and left) are frequently identical.
   b. The anterior communicating artery is located above the optic chiasm.
   c. Both arteries communicate via the anterior communicating artery.
   d. Both arteries first course medially to the internal carotid arteries.

4. What is the term used when the posterior cerebral arteries depend on the internal carotid artery for blood flow (at least partly)?
   a. normal PCA flow
   b. fetal origin of the PCA
   c. transposition of the PCA
   d. anomalous position of the PCA

5. Which of the following is a typical characteristic of a nonimaging transducer for transcranial Doppler?
   a. 1 to 2 MHz pulsed wave
   b. 1 to 2 MHz continuous wave
   c. >4 MHz pulsed wave
   d. >4 MHz continuous wave

6. What is the Doppler frequency range in standard duplex imaging system for transcranial imaging?
   a. 1 to 2 MHz
   b. 2 to 3 MHz
   c. 4 MHz
   d. >4MHz

7. What is the initial target vessel to be explored through the transtemporal acoustic window?
   a. ACA
   b. PCA
   c. MCA
   d. carotid siphon

8. What do the Lindegaard and the BA/VA ratios help categorize?
   a. distal ICA stenosis
   b. subarachnoid hemorrhaging
   c. dissections
   d. vasospasm

9. What does the relation MCA > ACA > PCA = BA = VA represent?
   a. relative flow velocities
   b. relative size of the vessels
   c. relative direction of flow in the vessels
   d. relation to the acoustic window

10. Which of the following is NOT a criterion used for the identification of vessels or vessel segments in the intracranial circulation?
    a. the direction of flow in relation to the transducer
    b. the diameter of the vessel
    c. the sample volume depth
    d. the vessel flow velocity

11. Which imaging technique creates a display that demonstrates flow intensity and direction in bands of color at multiple depths, creating a "road map" to follow signals from vessels?
    a. PW spectral Doppler
    b. CW spectral Doppler
    c. color Doppler
    d. power M-mode

12. Which of the following is NOT a primary diagnostic feature of the Doppler signals for evaluation of intracranial vessels?
    a. changes in various ratios from established criteria
    b. changes in velocity from established criteria
    c. changes in flow pulsatility from established standards
    d. changes in flow direction from established standards

13. Which collateral pathway will NOT show direct evidence of significant carotid artery disease?

    a. crossover collateral through ACoA

    b. posterior to anterior flow through PCoA

    c. leptomeningeal collateralization

    d. reversed ophthalmic artery

14. Which characteristic is NOT part of the five primary criteria used to identify intracranial arterial segment?

    a. flow direction

    b. pulsatility index

    c. sample volume depth

    d. window/approach used

15. A limited transcranial Doppler or transcranial duplex imaging exam could be ordered for all the following EXCEPT:

    a. evaluate for sickle cell anemia.

    b. monitor microembolism during endarterectomy.

    c. follow-up for vasospasm.

    d. evaluate single vessel patency.

16. Which statement regarding the use (and advantages) of audio signals during TCD and TCDI is FALSE?

    a. Nuances in signal can be heard before they can be seen on the Doppler spectrum.

    b. High-velocity signals could be missed by turbulent flow on the Doppler spectrum.

    c. Audio signals can help in redirecting the sonographer in the acquisition of Doppler spectrum.

    d. TCDI does not have audio capability.

17. Which of the following is the Atlas loop approach used for?

    a. Visualizing the internal carotid siphon.

    b. Visualizing the distal vertebral arteries.

    c. Obtaining data to characterize basilar artery vasospasm.

    d. Alternative window to the foramen magnum approach.

18. To ensure patient safety when using the transorbital approach, which technical setting should you always address?

    a. Decrease the acoustic intensity.

    b. Decrease the velocity scale.

    c. Increase the Doppler gain.

    d. Increase the color Doppler scale.

19. At a depth of approximately 65 mm from the transtemporal window, with a Doppler sample gate of 5 to 10 mm, you should obtain two Doppler spectra (one on each side of the baseline). What do these Doppler spectra correspond to?

    a. siphon/MCA

    b. right MCA/left MCA

    c. ACA/ACoA

    d. MCA/ACA

20. When is evidence of vasospasm usually seen following subarachnoid hemorrhaging?

    a. 3 to 4 days after the bleed started

    b. 6 to 8 days after the bleed started

    c. 2 to 4 weeks after the bleed started

    d. 6 to 8 weeks after the bleed started

Fill-in-the-Blank

1. On average, the center of the Circle of Willis is approximately the size of a _____.

2. The anterior intracranial arterial circulation is formed as a continuation of the _____.

3. The parasellar, genu, and supraclinoid segments are part of the _____.

4. The anterior inferior cerebellar and superior cerebellar arteries are branches of the _____.

5. From the transorbital window, the carotid siphon is identified at a depth of _____ mm.

6. The best acoustic window to insonate the vertebral and basilar arteries is through the _____.

7. The vessel identified through the transtemporal window at a depth of 65 mm with posterior and inferior rotation on the transducer is the _____.

8. Independently of the technique used (TCD or TCDI), the documentation of data obtained on intracranial arteries is based on _____.

9. All the arteries examined during a TCD or TCDI examination supply the brain except the _____.

10. When the transducer is placed 1.25 in below the mastoid process and posterior to the sternocleidomastoid muscle, the technique is called the _____ approach.

11. The Gosling index expresses the _____ of the Doppler signal.

12. The MCA mean velocity divided by the submandibular ICA mean velocity represents the calculation for the _____ ratio.

13. Ipsilateral increased velocities observed in the ACA and PCA with a significant stenosis or occlusion of the MCA is a result of _____ collateralization.

14. Evaluation of the MCA from a temporal window with a more posterior location will require aiming the transducer _____.

15. The most common mechanism of posterior circulation stroke, usually of cardiac origin, is _____.

16. Pediatric patients with _____ are recommended to have annual TCD screening to help prevent stroke.

17. For acute thrombosis, the _____ scale is used to classify changes that can occur rapidly with recanalization and re-occlusion in acute stroke.

18. Mean flow velocities in the MCA of >200 cm/s, a rapid daily rise in flow velocities and a hemispheric ratio ≥6.0 predicts the presence of significant _____.

19. A TCD signal that contains a very short or brief, high amplitude, unidirectional "snaps," "chirps," or "moans" indicates _____.

20. The finding that correlates with cerebral circulatory arrest is _____ in the TCD waveform.

Short Answer

1. With transcranial Doppler, why is spectral broadening unavoidable?

2. What are the main quantitative values used for diagnostic purposes in a transcranial exam?

3. Because of individual variations of the temporal window, how is this area subdivided?

IMAGE EVALUATION/PATHOLOGY

Review the images and answer the following questions.

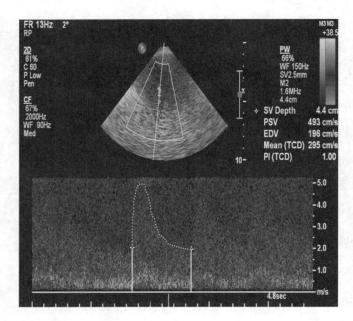

1. What do the Doppler spectrum profile and the flow velocities obtained in the right MCA suggest?

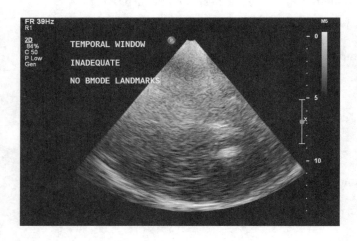

2. In this image, why would the examination be limited and diagnosis difficult? Which arteries of the circle of Willis would you not be able to obtain information for?

CASE STUDY

1. You are asked to evaluate a 25-year-old male, post–motor vehicle accident with a head injury, currently in critical condition in the intensive care unit. Your lab does not usually handle neurologic exams, so you do not have a set protocol for these exams. What would be the main consideration in this case? To set up an efficient protocol that will allow for sequential exams, the main arteries to monitor would be at a minimum. Which vessels would you assess, and what approach would you use? How would you set up your schedule to monitor this patient?

2. A 75-year-old female is seen for follow-up in the vascular lab. Previous exams have documented severe stenosis of the distal right internal carotid artery. The patient has remained mostly asymptomatic. In this examination, the result shows a complete occlusion of the right internal carotid artery. She still does not recall much change or symptoms. Her physician orders a transcranial study to assess the intracranial circulation. What collateral pathways could lead to this redistribution of flow? What would you expect the flow to be intracranially (particularly regarding direction of flow)?

PART FOUR

PERIPHERAL ARTERIAL

Indirect Assessment of Arterial Disease

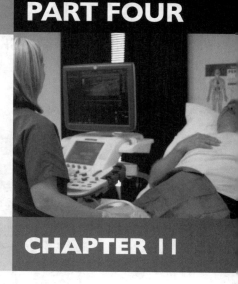

REVIEW OF GLOSSARY TERMS

Matching

Match the key terms with their definitions.

KEY TERMS

1. __b__ claudication
2. __a__ rest pain
3. __c__ ankle–brachial index
4. __f__ plethysmography
5. __e__ photoplethysmography
6. __d__ Raynaud's disease
7. __g__ thoracic outlet syndrome
8. __h__ Allen test

DEFINITION

a. Pain in the extremity without exercise or activity, thus, "at rest," can occur in the toes, foot, or ankle area

b. Pain in muscle groups brought on by exercise or activity that recedes with cessation of activity; can occur in the calf, thigh, and buttock

c. The ratio of ankle systolic pressure and brachial systolic pressure

d. Vasospasm of the digital arteries brought on by exposure to cold; can be caused by numerous etiologies

e. An indirect physiologic test that detects changes in back-scattered infrared light as an indicator of tissue perfusion

f. An indirect physiologic test that measures the change in volume or impedance in a whole body, organ, or limb

g. Compression of the brachial nerve plexus, subclavian artery, or subclavian vein at the region where these structures exit the thoracic cavity and course peripherally toward the arm

h. A series of maneuvers testing the digital perfusion of the hand while compressing and releasing the radial and ulnar arteries

ANATOMY AND PHYSIOLOGY REVIEW

Image Labeling

Complete the labels in the images that follow.

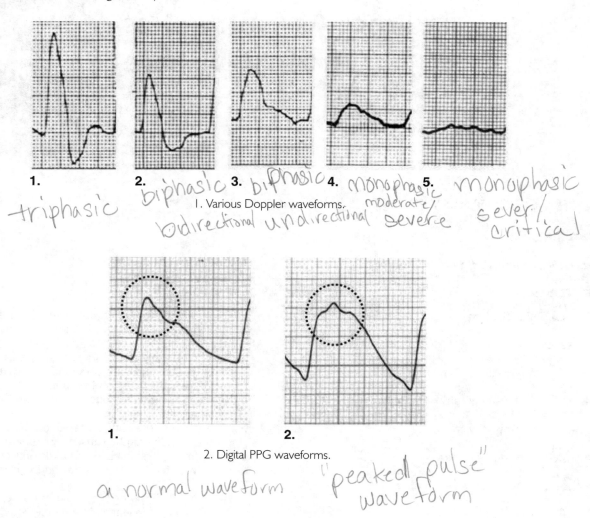

1. triphasic   2. biphasic bidirectional   3. biphasic undirectional   4. monophasic moderate severe   5. monophasic severe/critical

1. Various Doppler waveforms.

1. a normal waveform   2. "peaked pulse" waveform

2. Digital PPG waveforms.

CHAPTER REVIEW

Multiple Choice

Complete each question by circling the best answer.

1. Which method is most commonly used calculate ABI?
   a. The lowest pressure at the ankle to the lowest systolic pressure of the right or left brachial artery.
   b. The highest pressure at the ankle to the highest systolic pressure of the right or left brachial artery.
   c. The lowest pressure at the ankle to the highest systolic pressure of the right or left brachial artery.
   d. The highest pressure at the ankle to the lowest systolic pressure of the right or left brachial artery.

2. Which statement about intermittent claudication is FALSE?
   a. Pain with exercise is relieved by rest.
   b. It can be asymptomatic at rest.
   c. ABI values are generally between 0.5 and 1.3.
   d. ABI value can never be greater than 1.3.

3. Which statement regarding the importance of early assessment of the presence of PAD is FALSE?
   a. Patients are at increased risk for cardiovascular mortality.
   b. Patients are at increased risk for cardiovascular morbidity.
   c. Patients will eventually require an amputation.
   d. PAD is a marker for systemic arterial damage.

4. Progression of PAOD can be established on follow-up of patients by physical examination and clinical history because the patient may describe all the following EXCEPT:
   a. diminution of walking distance.
   b. increase of recovery time.
   c. skin and nails changes.
   d. resolution of pain by changing position.

5. Severe PAOD can be suspected with all the following EXCEPT:
   a. leg pain while sitting.
   b. skin discoloration and scaling.
   c. claudication pain after less than 50-ft walk.
   d. constant forefoot pain.

6. Thoracic outlet syndrome can include all the following presentations EXCEPT:
   a. pain with arm in neutral position.
   b. neurologic pain.
   c. edema of the arm and forearm.
   d. pain with arm elevated above head.

7. The techniques commonly used for indirect testing of arterial perfusion in the thigh and leg include all the following EXCEPT:
   a. plethysmography.
   b. photoplethysmography.
   c. Doppler waveforms analysis.
   d. segmental systolic pressure.

8. To ensure accuracy of data, particularly for recording of segmental systolic pressures, how long should the patient be allowed to rest?
   a. 5 to 10 minutes
   b. 10 to 15 minutes
   c. 20 minutes
   d. does not need to rest

9. What is the appropriate size for a blood pressure cuff to be used on an extremity to ensure accuracy of data obtained for systolic pressure determination?
   a. a 12-cm wide cuff at the upper arm
   b. a 10-cm wide cuff at the ankle
   c. between 10% and 15% wider than the diameter of the limb segment
   d. 20% wider than the diameter of the limb segment

10. All the following can result in inaccurate systolic pressure measurements in the lower extremities EXCEPT:
    a. the cuff is too narrow.
    b. the deflation rate is too fast.
    c. the limb segment is elevated above the heart.
    d. the dorsalis pedis artery is used to listen to the signal.

11. What will the use of a 4-cuff versus a 3-cuff method to estimate arterial disease in the lower extremities help determine?
    a. whether disease is present at the distal femoral level.
    b. whether disease is present at the proximal femoral level.
    c. whether disease is present at the iliofemoral level.
    d. whether disease is present at the popliteal level.

12. Which of the following is clear diagnostic criteria to estimate disease between two limb segments when using systolic pressure determination?

    a. A drop of more than 30 mm Hg between the proximal and immediate distal segment.

    b. An increase of more than 30 mm Hg between the proximal and immediate distal segment.

    c. A drop of 50 mm Hg between the proximal and immediate distal segment.

    d. An increase of 50 mm Hg between the proximal and immediate distal segment.

13. Which of the following is NOT a common method to induce symptoms with exercise in a patient suspected to have arterial insufficiency but relatively normal results at rest?

    a. Using a treadmill for walking with a set protocol.

    b. Having the patient walk at own pace until symptoms occur.

    c. Having the patient perform heel raises until symptoms occur.

    d. Raising the limb above the heart while the patient is supine on the exam table.

14. Which of the following is NOT one of the main advantages of pulse volume recording (PVR)?

    a. Records overall segment perfusion.

    b. Can give data even with calcified arteries.

    c. Is easy and quick to perform.

    d. Provides quantitative values.

15. What is the most convenient (and reliable) technique to obtain digital pressures while using a small digital cuff?

    a. PVR

    b. PPG

    c. CW Doppler

    d. PW Doppler

16. What is the most convenient technique to record changes of arterial insufficiency with thoracic outlet syndrome with a specific (and sometimes tailored) set of maneuvers?

    a. PVR on a limb segment

    b. CW Doppler at the brachial artery

    c. pressure recordings at the brachial artery

    d. PPG on a digit

17. What is the typical skin color changes (in the hands and fingers) associated with Raynaud's disease from room temperature to exposure to cold temperature and ending with rewarming?

    a. white, blue, red

    b. red, blue, white

    c. blue, white, red

    d. blue, red, white

18. The Allen test should be performed before all the following procedures EXCEPT:

    a. creation of an arteriovenous fistula.

    b. creation of a dialysis access.

    c. harvest of the cephalic vein for bypass.

    d. harvest of the radial artery for a coronary bypass.

19. The Allen test is typically performed by placing a PPG sensor on the middle or index finger to record digit perfusion while:

    a. the radial and ulnar arteries are compressed concomitantly.

    b. the radial and ulnar arteries are compressed sequentially.

    c. the radial artery is compressed individually.

    d. the ulnar artery is compressed individually.

20. Using PPG sensor on a digit demonstrating signs of increased vasospasm from primary Raynaud's disease, what characteristic will the waveform typically display?

    a. a peaked pulse on the anacrotic portion

    b. an anacrotic notch in late diastole

    c. a dicrotic notch in systole

    d. a dicrotic notch in diastole

Fill-in-the-Blank

1. Most often, symptoms of arterial disease are described as "intermittent" claudication because the symptoms occur only while active.

2. Symptoms observed or described with intermittent claudication can determine the site of disease because the disease is distal to the site of symptoms.

3. Lower extremity symptoms that require sitting and/or spinal flexure to relieve is usually associated with _Stenosis spinal_.

4. Elevation pallor and dependent rubor is usually observed with ___severe___ arterial disease.

5. The cause of primary Raynaud's disease is __idropathic__.

6. PAOD in the upper extremities occurs in __< 5%__ of all cases.

7. The ideal positioning of patients for indirect arterial testing should take great care that all extremities are not elevated above __the heat__.

8. For recording of accurate segmental systolic pressures, it is important not only to ensure the cuff is appropriate sized for the limb segment but also to allow the patient to ___rest___ before beginning the exam.

9. An ideal cuff deflation rate for accurately determining the return of Doppler signal when measuring systolic pressure at any segment should be approximately __3 mm/Hg /sec__

10. The lowest limit of an ABI to be considered within normal range at rest is __0.9__.

11. A change in ABI of __0.15__ between repeat studies indicates a significant change associated with worsening of PAOD.

12. When recording pressures from sites proximal to the ankle, the vessel (PTA or DPA) with the __systolic__ pressure is used to obtain the Doppler signal.

13. Under normal conditions (absence of disease), the high-thigh pressure using a 4-cuff method will usually be at least _____ greater than the normal brachial pressure.

14. In the upper extremities, using segmental pressure as diagnostic criteria, significant disease will be likely when a drop of at least ___30___ is recorded between two consecutive segments (from proximal to immediately distal segment).

15. ABIs returning to resting values more than 10 minutes postexercise are a good indication of __disease__.

16. Independently of the increasing discussion about the "correct" nomenclature to be used to describe continuous-wave (CW) Doppler waveforms, a normal CW Doppler waveform from an artery of the lower extremity should be ___triphasic___

17. The typical cuff inflation for segmental pulse volume recording (PVR) is _____.

18. CW Doppler and PVR waveforms analysis are examples of ___indirect___ criteria for the diagnosis of arterial disease.

19. A normal TBI (toe/brachial index) should be at least ___50___.

20. Testing for increased sensitivity to cold using immersion in ice water should only be used in patients with suspected __Raynauds disease__

Short Answer

1. What are the characteristic features of intermittent claudication that distinguishes it from other causes of lower extremity pain?

2. What is the typical protocol used for treadmill exercise testing to assess for claudication symptoms?

3. What are the upper extremity positions used when testing for thoracic outlet syndrome?

4. Why is normal resting systolic pressure higher at the ankle than at the brachial (without technical errors)?

5. What are the typical contraindications to exercise in determining the severity of arterial insufficiency in a patient with a relatively normal test at rest?

IMAGE EVALUATION/PATHOLOGY

Review the images and answer the following questions.

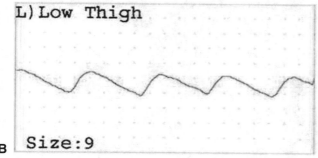

A   Size:9

B   Size:9

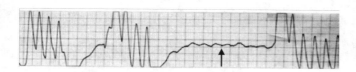

1. What technique were most likely use to obtain these waveforms?

   PVR

2. To what does the "size" (noted as size "9" here) relate?

   cuff size

3. Based solely on these images, where is the primary lesion?

4. This image was obtained from a patient sent to the vascular lab for assessment before harvesting of the radial artery for coronary bypass grafting. What is the name of the test being performed here?

   Allen's test

5. Based on the results of this test that the arrow shows the results with compression of the radial artery, what would you conclude?

   positive Allen's test

CASE STUDY

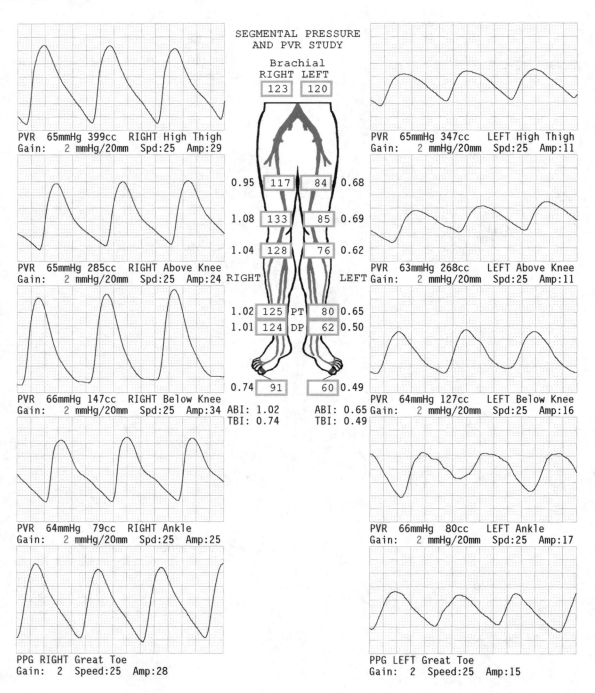

SEGMENTAL PRESSURE
AND PVR STUDY

Brachial
RIGHT LEFT
123   120

PVR 65mmHg 399cc RIGHT High Thigh
Gain: 2 mmHg/20mm Spd:25 Amp:29

PVR 65mmHg 347cc LEFT High Thigh
Gain: 2 mmHg/20mm Spd:25 Amp:11

0.95 117   84 0.68

1.08 133   85 0.69

1.04 128   76 0.62

PVR 65mmHg 285cc RIGHT Above Knee
Gain: 2 mmHg/20mm Spd:25 Amp:24

PVR 63mmHg 268cc LEFT Above Knee
Gain: 2 mmHg/20mm Spd:25 Amp:11

RIGHT   LEFT

1.02 125 PT   80 0.65
1.01 124 DP   62 0.50

PVR 66mmHg 147cc RIGHT Below Knee
Gain: 2 mmHg/20mm Spd:25 Amp:34

PVR 64mmHg 127cc LEFT Below Knee
Gain: 2 mmHg/20mm Spd:25 Amp:16

0.74   91   60 0.49

ABI: 1.02   ABI: 0.65
TBI: 0.74   TBI: 0.49

PVR 64mmHg 79cc RIGHT Ankle
Gain: 2 mmHg/20mm Spd:25 Amp:25

PVR 66mmHg 80cc LEFT Ankle
Gain: 2 mmHg/20mm Spd:25 Amp:17

PPG RIGHT Great Toe
Gain: 2 Speed:25 Amp:28

PPG LEFT Great Toe
Gain: 2 Speed:25 Amp:15

1. You are asked to interpret an indirect arterial assessment on a patient for suspected arterial insufficiency from one of your staff technologists. The patient is in the intensive care unit and unresponsive. The patient was recently admitted, and aside from the physician's note stating decreased pulses in the left lower extremity, you have no other records available.

   The record shows an ABI on the left of 0.65 (at rest) with an ABI on the right of 1.02, and the waveforms as seen on the image. What technique was used to obtain waveforms in this exam? How do you know? What do the results suggest (based on the analysis of waveforms and ABI)? Were there technical errors? If so, explain.

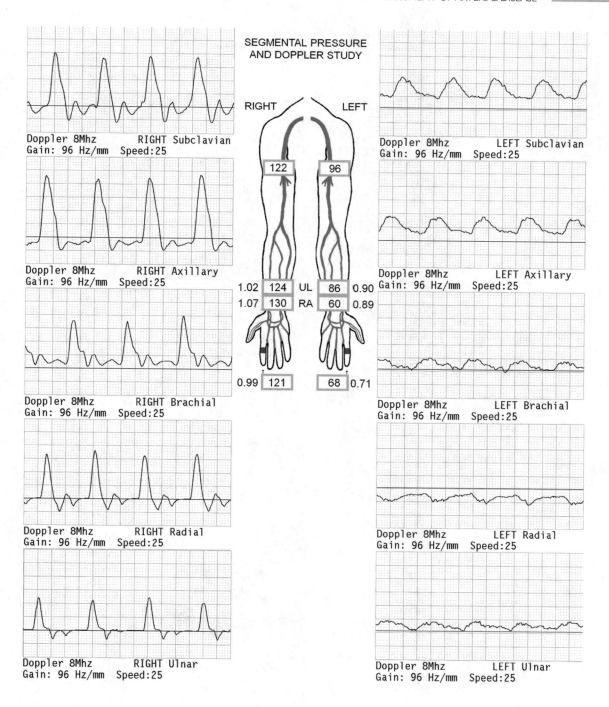

SEGMENTAL PRESSURE
AND DOPPLER STUDY

RIGHT   LEFT

Doppler 8Mhz RIGHT Subclavian	Doppler 8Mhz LEFT Subclavian
Gain: 96 Hz/mm Speed:25	Gain: 96 Hz/mm Speed:25
Doppler 8Mhz RIGHT Axillary	Doppler 8Mhz LEFT Axillary
Gain: 96 Hz/mm Speed:25	Gain: 96 Hz/mm Speed:25
Doppler 8Mhz RIGHT Brachial	Doppler 8Mhz LEFT Brachial
Gain: 96 Hz/mm Speed:25	Gain: 96 Hz/mm Speed:25
Doppler 8Mhz RIGHT Radial	Doppler 8Mhz LEFT Radial
Gain: 96 Hz/mm Speed:25	Gain: 96 Hz/mm Speed:25
Doppler 8Mhz RIGHT Ulnar	Doppler 8Mhz LEFT Ulnar
Gain: 96 Hz/mm Speed:25	Gain: 96 Hz/mm Speed:25

122   96

1.02 124 UL 86 0.90
1.07 130 RA 60 0.89

0.99 121   68 0.71

2. A patient presents to the vascular lab for an upper extremity indirect arterial evaluation, with an additional request to assess for thoracic outlet syndrome. The patient notes left arm pain that seems to be related to use but not necessarily position. The left radial pulse is noted to be diminished when compared to the right.

   The results of the segmental pressure and Doppler waveform study are presented in this image. What do these findings suggest? Would TOS testing be appropriate in this individual? Why or why not? Are there other vessels outside the upper extremity that might benefit from duplex evaluation based on these findings?

left is abnormal, left proximal disease

Duplex Ultrasound of Lower Extremity Arteries

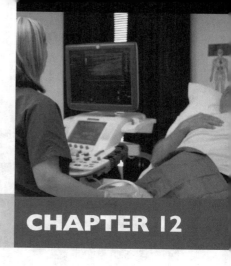

CHAPTER 12

REVIEW OF GLOSSARY OF TERMS

Matching

Match the key terms with their definitions.

KEY TERMS

1. _____ duplex arteriography

2. _____ contrast arteriography

3. _____ plaque

4. _____ aneurysm

DEFINITION

a. A radiologic imaging technique performed using ionizing radiation to provide detailed arterial system configuration and pathology information

b. A localized dilation of an artery involving all three layers of the arterial wall

c. Ultrasound imaging of the arterial system performed to identify atherosclerotic disease and other arterial pathology, providing a detailed map of the arterial system evaluated

d. The deposit of fatty material within the vessel walls, which is characteristic of atherosclerosis

ANATOMY AND PHYSIOLOGY REVIEW

Image Labeling

Complete the labels in the images that follow.

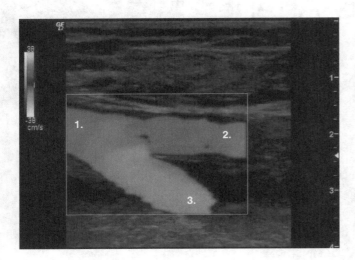

1. Label the vessels in the image.

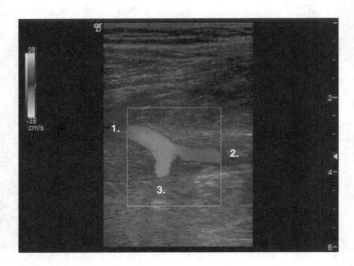

2. Label the vessels in the image.

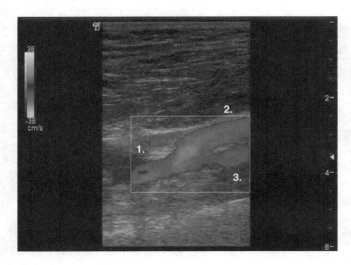

3. Label the vessels in the image.

CHAPTER REVIEW

Multiple Choice

Complete each question by circling the best answer.

1. What is the main technical limitation in the routine use of duplex ultrasound instead of contrast angiography to visualize the arteries of the lower extremities due to?
   a. Most plaque will be calcified.
   b. Most equipment does not have that imaging capacity.
   c. Most sonographers are not trained to obtain diagnostic data.
   d. Most physicians are not trained to interpret data.

2. On a posterior approach of the popliteal fossa, what is the branch identified on the anterior aspect of the image in relation to the popliteal artery?
   a. the anterior tibial artery
   b. a geniculate artery
   c. a gastrocnemius artery
   d. the tibioperoneal trunk

3. Which artery is best visualized by a posterolateral approach at the level of the calf?
   a. the posterior tibial artery
   b. the peroneal artery
   c. the popliteal artery
   d. the tibioperoneal trunk

4. Which method represents good practice to thoroughly evaluate arterial disease in the lower extremities when using B-mode to view the vessel?
   a. Viewing in sagittal only
   b. Viewing in transverse only
   c. Moving from medial to lateral
   d. Using both transverse and longitudinal planes

5. What is the primary tool to evaluate disease of the lower extremity arteries using duplex ultrasound (at the exception of aneurysm)?
   a. aliasing on color Doppler
   b. B-mode image
   c. color display with power Doppler
   d. peak systolic velocity

6. How is the velocity ratio (Vr) calculated?
   a. PSV at stenosis divided by PSV proximal to stenosis.
   b. PSV proximal to stenosis divided by PSV at stenosis.
   c. PSV at stenosis divided by PSV distal to stenosis.
   d. PSV distal to stenosis divided by PSV at stenosis.

7. Which of the following is NOT a consideration when assessing for the possibility of treatment of an arterial lesion by angioplasty or stenting (or both)?
   a. size of the artery
   b. position of branches
   c. length of the stenosis
   d. location of the stenosis

8. Why does duplex ultrasound have an advantage over contrast angiography for the examination of vessel walls?
   a. The plaque thickness can be measured.
   b. The plaque characteristics can be determined.
   c. The wall thickness can be measured.
   d. The remaining lumen can be measured.

9. Which of the following is a main pitfall of duplex ultrasound (in general) in examining arterial disease?
   a. flow at velocities less than 20 cm/s
   b. flow at velocities over 400 cm/s
   c. length of occluded segment
   d. collateral vessels

10. When using duplex ultrasound to record slow flow (<20 cm/s) in an arterial segment, which of the following adjustments would NOT be useful?
    a. Decrease the PRF.
    b. Use a low wall filter.
    c. Increase the persistence of color.
    d. Decrease the Doppler gain.

11. When assessing the appearance of a plaque on a grayscale image, what might an irregular plaque surface indicate?
    a. stable plaque unlikely to rupture
    b. an area of necrosis
    c. an area of ulceration
    d. thrombus formation on top of the plaque

12. Why is reporting the presence of a partial thrombus in an aneurysm important?
    a. Partial thrombus may not be visible on contrast angiography.
    b. Pieces of thrombus can embolize.
    c. The lumen may not be enlarged.
    d. It will likely proceed to an acute occlusion.

13. When can a greater than 70% stenosis in any arteries of the lower extremities be safely inferred?
    a. The PSV is half distal to the stenosis.
    b. The PSV is doubled at the stenosis.
    c. The Vr is equal to or greater than 2.
    d. The Vr is equal to or greater than 3.

14. How is low-resistance blood flow characterized on a Doppler spectrum?
    a. antegrade flow throughout diastole
    b. antegrade flow in systole only
    c. retrograde flow in systole
    d. sharp downstroke in early diastole

15. Which of the following is NOT a potential pathologic finding when the Doppler spectrum of an artery of the lower extremity displays low-resistance characteristics?
    a. arteriovenous fistula
    b. postreactive hyperemia
    c. cellulitis
    d. trauma

16. Doppler spectra with a characteristic low-resistance outline may be seen distal to a hemodynamically significant stenosis. What will the Doppler spectra also display?
    a. delay on the downstroke in systole
    b. delay on the upstroke in systole
    c. retrograde flow in diastole
    d. retrograde flow in systole

17. What characteristic outline will Doppler spectra in an arterial segment proximal to a hemodynamically significant stenosis or an occlusion have?
    a. no flow in diastole
    b. no flow in systole
    c. retrograde flow in diastole
    d. retrograde flow in systole

18. Which of the following is NOT a factor typically associated with the need to perform contrast angiography after a limited duplex ultrasound of the arterial system?
    a. high infrapopliteal vessel calcification
    b. limb-threatening ischemia
    c. female gender
    d. older age

19. Why is the use of contrast angiography in diabetic patients particularly worrisome?
    a. ionizing radiation
    b. nephrotoxic agents
    c. poor visualization of calcified segments
    d. poor visualization of low flow

20. What aspects of duplex ultrasound assessment of the lower extremity arteries allow better estimation of the true hemodynamic significance of an arterial lesion, when compared to contrast angiography?
    a. Doppler spectrum analysis and color Doppler
    b. Doppler spectrum analysis only
    c. power and color Doppler
    d. flow velocities and velocity ratio

Fill-in-the-Blank

1. Conditions and risk factors for which patients are referred for duplex ultrasound of the lower extremity arteries are _____ as those for indirect physiologic testing.

2. The below-knee segment of the popliteal artery is best examined through a _____ approach.

3. Most arteries of the lower extremity can be examined by duplex ultrasound using a _____ approach.

4. The two arteries or arterial segments, which cannot be well examined with duplex ultrasound via a medial approach, are the popliteal artery and _____.

5. The superficial femoral artery typically changes name to become the popliteal artery as the vessel exits the _____.

6. On a posterior approach of the upper calf, the artery branching off the popliteal artery deep to the popliteal artery is most likely the _____.

7. In general, color and power Doppler's primary advantage is for _____ and tracking of the vessels.

8. When an occlusion is discovered during duplex assessment of the lower extremity arteries, documentation of where the vessel is _____ by collateral flow is useful to the vascular surgeon.

9. To evaluate the dorsalis pedis and distal posterior tibial arteries adequately, a sonographer should be particularly careful with the _____ from the transducer.

10. Duplex ultrasound is superior to contrast angiography in determining a suitable site for the distal anastomosis of a graft because it can detect the _____ area of the vessel wall.

11. Using a lower frequency transducer to view the SFA at the adductor canal or the tibioperoneal trunk at the upper calf will reduce _____.

12. Determining/characterizing the "nature" of a plaque or wall thickening is important information a sonographer can convey to a surgeon because _____ through a calcified plaque is almost impossible.

13. Although the peak systolic velocity (PSV) is the primary measurement obtained, stenoses are classified based on _____.

14. Using duplex ultrasound instead of contrast angiography in patients with severe-to-critical limb ischemia is recommended because the examination with duplex is more _____.

15. A vessel is considered aneurysmal if the diameter is _____ times greater than the more proximal segment.

16. Very low flow, particularly to assess the patency of possible outflow vessels, is more easily achieved with duplex ultrasound than with contrast angiography with the use of _____.

17. When assessing the lower extremity arterial system with duplex ultrasound, only the first few centimeters of the _____ artery are evaluated.

18. Distal to a hemodynamically significant stenosis, the Doppler waveform demonstrates poststenotic _____.

19. At a measured diameter of 1.1 cm, a common femoral artery would be considered _____, whereas a popliteal artery that measures 1.1 cm would be considered _____.

20. As compared to contrast arteriography, duplex ultrasound allows direct visualization of the entire artery and not just the _____.

Short Answer

1. What are the symptoms associated with acute arterial ischemia?

2. Why is it important for the vascular technologist to provide as much information as possible regarding arterial anatomy and disease to the referring physician?

3. What are the main advantages of duplex arteriography, especially as compared to contrast arteriography?

IMAGE EVALUATION/PATHOLOGY

Review the images and answer the following questions.

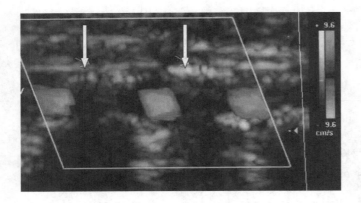

1. What area do the arrows point to?

2. How would you substantiate the answer to the previous question?

3. Is stenosis likely at the area not adequately visualized? Explain.

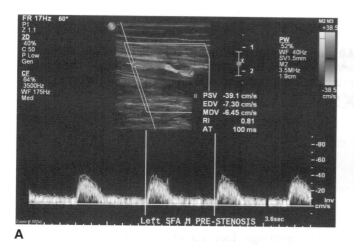

A

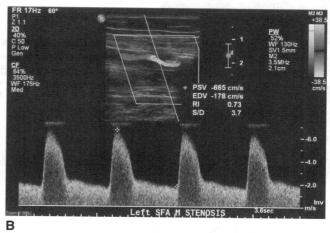

B

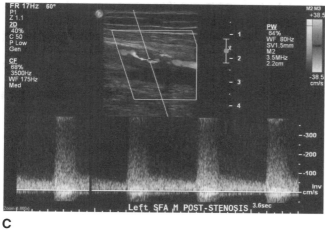

C

4. What do each of these waveforms demonstrate?

5. What percent stenosis is present in the above images?

ANATOMY AND PHYSIOLOGY REVIEW

Image Labeling

Complete the labels in the image that follows.

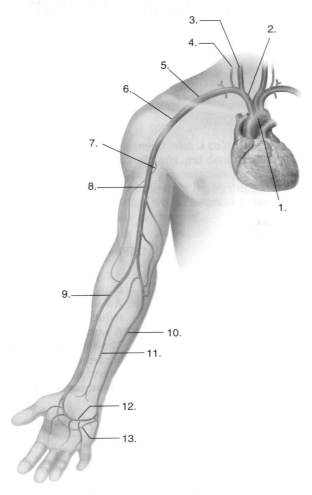

1. Principle upper extremity arteries.

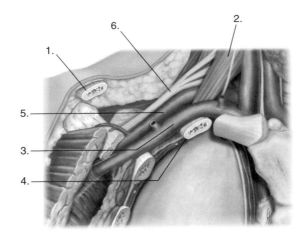

2. Anatomy of the thoracic outlet.

CHAPTER REVIEW

Multiple Choice

Complete each question by circling the best answer.

1. What percentage of extremity peripheral arterial disease do upper extremity arterial diseases represent?
   a. 5%
   b. 15%
   c. 20%
   d. 50%

2. Which of the following is NOT a prominent etiology of arterial diseases in the upper extremities?
   a. mechanical obstruction or compression at the thoracic outlet
   b. embolism from various sources (including the heart)
   c. vasoconstriction of digital arteries
   d. diffuse atherosclerosis of the axillary or brachial artery

3. What is a dilated segment of the proximal descending aorta which may give rise to the takeoff of an aberrant subclavian artery?
   a. Ortner syndrome
   b. thoracic outlet syndrome
   c. Raynaud's syndrome
   d. Kommerell's diverticulum

4. Which of the following is NOT a common site for compression of the subclavian artery?
   a. compression between the first rib and scalene muscle
   b. compression between the clavicle and first rib
   c. compression by the brachial plexus
   d. compression by the pectoralis minor

5. Which of the following is NOT a potential consequence of compression of the subclavian artery at the thoracic outlet?
   a. thrombosis
   b. embolism
   c. stenosis
   d. aneurysm

6. Injury of what artery may result in hypothenar hammer syndrome?
   a. the radial artery at the wrist
   b. the interosseous artery at mid forearm
   c. the ulnar artery at the wrist
   d. the posterior branch of the radial artery

7. Which arteries do the sternal notch window, and the infraclavicular and supraclavicular approaches, all used to visualize?
   a. the subclavian arteries
   b. the vertebral arteries
   c. the common carotid arteries
   d. the axillary arteries

8. Under normal conditions, what is the flow-velocity range of the arteries in the forearm?
   a. 80 to 120 cm/s
   b. 40 to 60 cm/s
   c. 120 to 150 cm/s
   d. 10 to 20 cm/s

9. With what condition are aneurysms of the subclavian arteries often associated?
   a. vasospasm
   b. injury or trauma
   c. thoracic outlet syndrome
   d. Raynaud's disease

10. What is the landmark that marks the transition from the axillary artery to the brachial artery?
    a. superior border of the first rib
    b. inferolateral border of the teres major muscle
    c. posterolateral border of the pectoralis major muscle
    d. lateral margin of the first rib

11. How is primary Raynaud's syndrome distinguished from secondary Raynaud's syndrome or Raynaud's phenomenon?
    a. There are underlying diseases.
    b. There are no underlying diseases.
    c. There is no distinction.
    d. The symptoms are different.

12. Although rare, digital artery occlusion from embolization may occur. Which of the following is NOT a predominant source of embolization?
    a. subclavian artery aneurysms
    b. stenosis of proximal upper extremity arteries
    c. fibromuscular diseases of arteries of the forearm
    d. thromboangiitis obliterans

13. To efficiently assess perfusion and/or vasospasm of digital arteries, how should one record waveforms obtained with PPG?
    a. pre- and postwarming of fingers
    b. pre- and postexercise
    c. pre- and post-cold immersion
    d. pre- and post-arm abduction

14. Compression of structures at the thoracic outlet may happen with all of the following EXCEPT:
    a. hypertrophy of the scalene muscle.
    b. hypertrophy of the pectoralis minor muscle.
    c. the presence of a cervical rib.
    d. the presence of abnormal fibrous bands.

15. Which statement regarding compression of the brachial plexus and vascular structures at the thoracic outlet is FALSE?
    a. Compression of either will give similar symptoms.
    b. Compression of either cannot be easily confirmed by provocative maneuvers.
    c. Compression of both often occurs concomitantly.
    d. Confirmation of neural symptoms is best done by electromyography (EMG).

16. How is "arterial minor" form of thoracic outlet syndrome defined?
    a. Intermittent compression of the subclavian artery when arm is in neutral position.
    b. Significant compression of the subclavian artery by clavicle.
    c. Intermittent compression of the subclavian when arm is raised overhead.
    d. Significant compression of the subclavian artery by first rib.

17. Which condition is associated with significant stenosis or occlusion of arteries of the arm and/or forearm from atherosclerosis?
    a. diabetes and/or renal failure
    b. coronary artery disease
    c. peripheral arterial disease
    d. systemic diseases

18. A 47-year-old male smoker presents to the vascular lab with ulcerations of his fingertips. What disease process should be suspected in this patient?
    a. steal syndrome from small vessels disease
    b. Buerger's disease
    c. Raynaud's syndrome
    d. embolism from subclavian artery aneurysm

19. Which form of arterial inflammation can affect the ophthalmic artery as well as the subclavian or axillary?
    a. Takayasu's arteritis
    b. Raynaud's phenomenon
    c. Buerger's disease
    d. giant cell arteritis

20. What is the most significant difference between giant cell arteritis and Takayasu's disease when both affect the subclavian artery?
    a. the age of the patient
    b. the gender of the patient
    c. the health of the patient
    d. the body habitus of the patient

Fill-in-the-Blank

1. The _____ artery is the first major branch of the aortic arch and divides into the right common carotid and subclavian arteries.

2. On the left, the _____ artery arises directly from the aortic arch in 4% to 6% of patients.

3. The artery resting between the biceps muscle anteriorly and triceps muscle posteriorly is the _____ artery.

4. The artery, which lies deep to the pectoralis major and minor, is the _____ artery.

5. A high takeoff occurs most commonly as a variant of the _____ artery.

6. The interosseous artery commonly takes off from the _____ artery.

7. The evaluation of the axillary artery by duplex is often accomplished with the arm in the _____ position.

8. Using the sternal notch window, the origin of the subclavian artery is usually first identified with color Doppler in a _____ view.

9. With Doppler, all arteries in the upper extremities should, under normal conditions, exhibit _____ resistance.

10. To assist in the visualization of the relatively small caliber arteries in the forearm, the sonographer may use _____ of the arm to increase blood flow.

11. The most common systemic condition resulting in secondary Raynaud's syndrome is _____.

12. Digital artery necrosis associated with Raynaud's symptoms will rarely be seen with _____ Raynaud's syndrome.

13. Provocative maneuvers demonstrating subclavian artery compression at the thoracic outlet may occur in 20% of _____ individuals.

14. Unilateral digital ischemia should prompt the sonographer to look for a source of _____ from more proximal arteries.

15. Duplex ultrasound has been shown to be an effective means of evaluating for upper extremity _____, even though computed tomographic arteriography or direct surgical exploration is currently the standard of care.

16. Clinically, significant stenosis or occlusion of upper extremity arteries from atherosclerosis is typically confined to the _____ artery.

17. Symptoms of fever, malaise, arthralgia, and myalgia are not uncommon in the _____ phase of Takayasu's disease.

18. Immunosuppressant and anti-inflammatory medications are the primary treatment for several forms of _____.

19. A definite diagnosis for Buerger's disease is best achieved with _____.

20. When evaluating a vessel for aneurysm, it is important to visualize in a true _____ plane to not falsely overestimate the diameter.

Short Answer

1. What is a retroesophageal subclavian artery? What, if any, symptoms may the patient have as a result?

2. How are the vertebral arteries distinguished from the thyrocervical and costocervical trunks?

3. While there are not accepted velocity criteria to determine the degree of stenosis in the upper extremity arteries, what are the general guidelines correlating with >50% stenosis?

4. When trauma occurs in the upper extremity, what pathologic findings should the vascular technologist be concerned about, and are often visualized on the B-mode image?

IMAGE EVALUATION/PATHOLOGY

Review the images and answer the following questions.

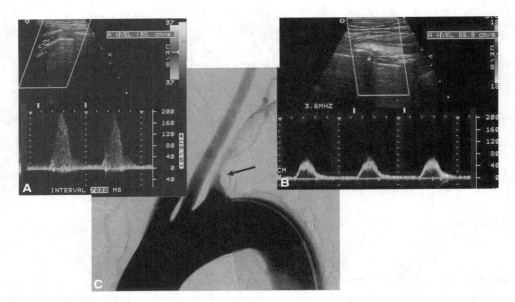

1. Which of the Doppler spectrums (A) or (B) would best represent what could be expected at the area designated by the arrow on angiogram (C)?

2. Which artery is showing pathology in these images?

3. Where could you find Doppler spectrum (B)—distal or proximal to the stenosis?

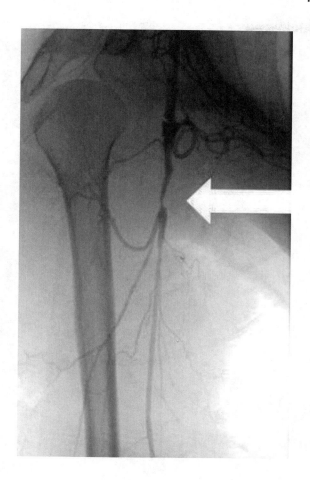

4. Based on the landmarks visible on this angiogram, the arrow points to a defect in which vessel?

5. What would you expect to see with corresponding Doppler and color Doppler on ultrasound?

CASE STUDY

1. A healthy 45-year-old female presents to the vascular lab (located in Vermont) in mid-February, with ischemic and color changes in several digits of her hands and feet. What should your initial questions focus on? She reveals that she is an avid skier and spends most of her free time "on the slopes." What do you expect the results of your exam to reveal?

2. A 25-year-old male working for the civil engineering department of the city presents with a pulsatile mass on the level of the medial aspect of the wrist extending slightly to the upper palm of his right hand. Small ischemic changes are also evident at the tip of the fourth and fifth fingers. What is the most probable cause for this presentation? What is the best test you could use for diagnosis in the vascular lab? What do you expect the results will reveal?

Ultrasound Assessment of Arterial Bypass Grafts

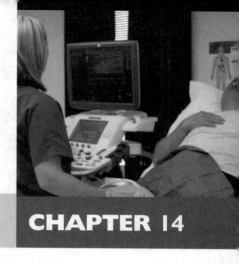

CHAPTER 14

REVIEW OF GLOSSARY OF TERMS

Matching

Match the key terms with their definitions.

KEY TERMS

1. _____ bypass

2. _____ graft

3. _____ in situ bypass

4. _____ anastomosis

5. _____ arteriovenous fistula

6. _____ hyperemia

DEFINITION

a. A conduit that can be prosthetic material or autogenous vein used to divert blood flow from one artery to another

b. A connection between an artery and a vein that was created because of surgery or by other iatrogenic means

c. A channel that diverts blood flow from one artery to another, usually done to shunt flow around an occluded portion of a vessel

d. The great saphenous vein is left in place in its normal anatomical position and used to create a diversionary channel for blood flow around an occluded artery

e. An increase in blood flow. This can occur following exercise. It can also occur following restoration of blood flow following periods of ischemia

f. A connection created surgically to connect two vessels that were formerly not connected

ANATOMY AND PHYSIOLOGY REVIEW

Image Labeling

Complete the labels in the images that follow.

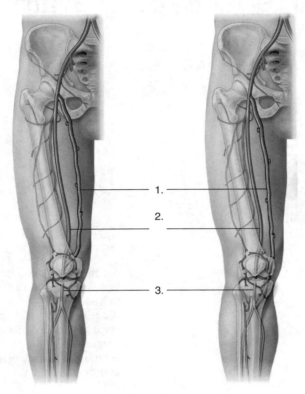

1. Types of vein bypass grafts.

CHAPTER REVIEW

Multiple Choice

Complete each question by circling the best answer.

1. Which of the following is NOT considered a method of assessment of a lower extremity infrainguinal by-pass graft?
   a. physical/clinical evaluation
   b. ankle to brachial index
   c. chemical blood chemistry panel
   d. plethysmography

2. Which veins would be typically used for an in situ bypass in the lower extremity?
   a. the cephalic vein
   b. the basilic vein
   c. the small saphenous vein
   d. the great saphenous vein

3. What is an advantage of synthetic grafts when compared to autogenous vein grafts?
   a. high thrombogenic potential
   b. low rate of early technical problems
   c. high rate of progressive stenosis at the inflow artery
   d. high long-term patency rate

4. Why are in situ infrainguinal bypass grafts using the great saphenous vein a common and preferred technique?
   a. There is a better match of vessel size at the in-flow and outflow.
   b. There is no need to lyze the valves.
   c. The branches of the great saphenous vein provide additional collateral.
   d. This allows for reverse flow.

5. What is the term to describe an autogenous vein graft in which the vein retains its original anatomical direction?
   a. reverse
   b. antegrade
   c. orthograde
   d. retrograde

6. Independent of the type of bypass graft used, where is the distal anastomosis typically located?
   a. distal to the disease
   b. proximal to the disease
   c. at the level of the popliteal artery
   d. at the level of the dorsalis pedis

7. Which of the following is NOT one of the main causes for early autogenous vein graft thrombosis (within the first 30 days)?
   a. underlying hypercoagulable state
   b. myointimal hyperplasia
   c. inadequate vein conduit
   d. inadequate run-off bed

8. After 24 months, what is the likely cause of stenosis in the inflow or outflow vessels?
   a. myointimal hyperplasia
   b. retained or improperly placed suture
   c. progression of atherosclerotic disease
   d. graft entrapment

9. At a minimum, which physiologic test should be included when assessing a lower extremity bypass graft?
   a. full segmental pressure exam with CW Doppler waveforms
   b. PVR waveforms only
   c. PVR waveforms with high thigh and below-knee pressures
   d. ankle-brachial index

10. Which artery is NOT commonly used as inflow for a bypass graft in the lower extremities?
    a. common femoral artery
    b. profunda femoris
    c. geniculate artery
    d. popliteal artery

11. Which transducer would allow optimal near-field imaging for the evaluation of a superficial, in situ vein graft?
    a. 2 to 3 MHz sector
    b. 3 to 5 MHz curvilinear
    c. 5 to 7 MHz linear
    d. 10 to 12 MHz linear

12. What view can be used for an initial rough scan of a bypass graft, including inflow and outflow, and may be helpful to identify tributaries of an in situ graft?
    a. sagittal
    b. coronal
    c. transverse
    d. long-axis

13. Which of the following is NOT a potential incidental finding related to the perigraft space?
    a. retained valve
    b. seroma
    c. hematoma
    d. abscesses

14. Where will myointimal hyperplasia in an autogenous vein graft typically occur?
    a. at the proximal anastomosis
    b. at the distal anastomosis
    c. at a site of previous valve sinus
    d. in the midgraft only

15. If an intimal flap or a dissection is present in a bypass graft, what is the typical cause?
    a. valve retention
    b. intraoperative technical problem
    c. fibrosis in the inflow artery
    d. aneurysms at the distal anastomosis

16. In synthetic aortofemoral or femoro-femoral grafts, where may pseudoaneurysms, while rare, occur?
    a. the midgraft
    b. anywhere along the length of the graft
    c. the proximal anastomosis
    d. the distal anastomosis

17. Arteriovenous fistula, occasionally seen in in situ bypass grafts, results from failure to ligate which of the following?
    a. the small saphenous vein
    b. a perforating vein
    c. a small arterial branch
    d. a defect at valve lysis

18. How is mean graft flow velocity calculated?
    a. Taking several measurements at the midgraft level.
    b. Averaging the velocities at the proximal and distal anastomoses.
    c. Averaging the velocities from the inflow and outflow arteries.
    d. Averaging three or four velocities from nonstenotic segments.

19. What is the first modality that should be used to examine a bypass graft?
    a. B-mode
    b. spectral Doppler
    c. color Doppler
    d. power Doppler

20. On follow-up of a bypass graft done 4 years ago, what may a Doppler spectrum displaying delay in systole indicate?
    a. technical defect at the anastomosis
    b. atherosclerotic stenosis at the inflow
    c. arteriovenous fistula within the graft
    d. imminent failure from distal occlusion

Fill-in-the-Blank

1. Duplex ultrasound has been shown to be reliable in the detection of significant pathology in infrainguinal bypass graft in _____ patients, before measurable changes in physiologic testing.

2. Combining physiologic study with duplex ultrasound for the assessment of an infrainguinal bypass graft is important for the detection of significant pathology and the evaluation of _____.

3. Types of bypass grafts can be categorized based on the material used for the graft and _____ employed.

4. Vein grafts have a longer patency rate than synthetic grafts (independently of the location) because vein grafts are less _____.

5. Types of materials used for infrainguinal bypass grafts include autogenous veins, synthetic materials, and _____.

6. Within the first 30 days of the perioperative period following the implantation of a bypass graft, the most common problems are _____ problems.

7. In the 1- to 24-month postoperative period, 75% of graft revisions are done for stenoses at the proximal or distal _____.

8. To document a stenosis within a bypass graft most completely, the PSV and EDV proximal, within, and distal to the stenosis should be noted, as well as poststenotic _____.

9. To ensure accurate documentation during a follow-up for a bypass graft, it is important for the sonographer to be familiar with the type and location of the bypass and, therefore, refer to _____.

10. Twenty-four months after a bypass graft has been performed, the main cause of failure will be _____, primarily in the inflow and outflow arteries.

11. During follow-up exams of bypass graft using comparison of flow velocities for diagnostic purpose, an effort should be made to obtain the velocities in the same location, as well as with the same _____ as previously employed.

12. When evaluating the distal anastomosis and outflow artery of a bypass graft, a(n) _____ in peak systolic velocity in the outflow artery can be encountered because the artery may have a smaller caliber.

13. Within the vein conduit, the two most common image abnormalities that are observed are _____ and _____.

14. Color Doppler can be useful in the evaluation of a bypass for defects; however, care must be taken because color can also _____ small wall defects or other pathology.

15. Although located in the lower extremities, Doppler spectrum in a bypass graft can display _____-resistance characteristics, often due to hyperemia or arteriovenous fistula.

16. A blunted, monophasic spectral Doppler pattern with zero diastolic flow typically indicates _____.

17. A decrease of mean graft flow velocity of more than _____ from previous exam is indicative of potential failure of the graft.

18. A velocity ratio of 3.5 and a PSV >300 cm/s is consistent with a _____% stenosis.

19. A tunneled PTFE femoral to popliteal graft will be _____ than an in situ graft.

20. To examine the distal anastomosis and outflow of a femoral to dorsalis pedis bypass graft, one may opt to select a transducer with _____ frequency.

Short Answer

1. What is an important consideration when choosing autogenous veins for infrainguinal bypass grafts in a reverse position?

2. What are the indications for a duplex ultrasound evaluation of a bypass graft outside the routine surveillance schedule?

3. What is the typical surveillance schedule of an autogenous vein bypass graft? When might this schedule be altered?

4. What is the minimum suggested documentation of a bypass graft on duplex ultrasound assessment?

IMAGE EVALUATION/PATHOLOGY

Review the images and answer the following questions.

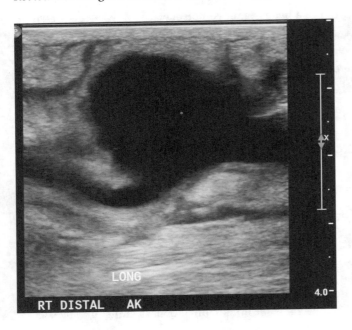

1. What pathology can be seen in the figure?

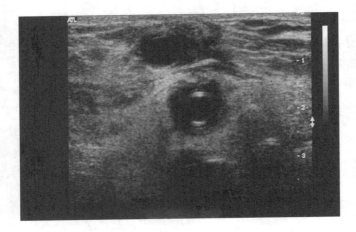

2. What does this image suggest?

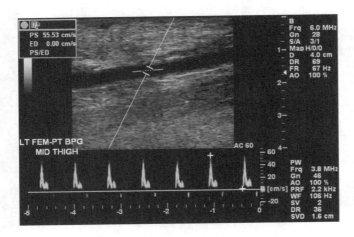

3. What does the Doppler waveform pattern seen in this image seem to suggest?

CASE STUDY

1. A 75-year-old male with a long-standing history of cardiovascular disease and vascular reconstruction in the lower extremities presents with a pulsatile mass in the right inguinal area. The history of vascular reconstruction includes an aortobifemoral bypass graft and a left femoral to popliteal bypass graft. What are two possibilities to explain the presence of the pulsatile mass?

2. An 81-year-old female presents to the vascular lab with a cold right foot and evidence of ulceration on several digits of the right foot. She is not one of your regular patients. You do not have any records on this patient, and she cannot recall what was done or when, but you see some scars on the medial aspect of the leg, suggesting that a bypass graft may have been done. What should your initial test/assessment be?

   After your initial assessment, you decide to use duplex ultrasound to get an idea of what was done. Slightly below the inguinal ligament, you see the takeoff of a "vessel" with bright white, double-lined walls and flow with spectral and color Doppler. What does this finding suggest?

   You cannot assess the graft further than 1 to 2 cm distal to the anastomosis, so you sample the proximal portion of the graft and attempt to find the distal anastomosis or outflow. You obtain a Doppler signal at the popliteal artery. The Doppler spectrum in the proximal graft shows PSV of 130 cm/s with no diastolic flow and very sharp but narrow waveforms. The Doppler spectrum at the popliteal artery shows delay in systole and a PSV of 11 cm/s with diastolic flow. What can you infer from these data?

Duplex Ultrasound Testing Following Peripheral Endovascular Arterial Intervention

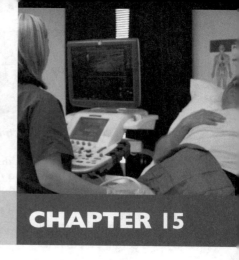

CHAPTER 15

REVIEW OF GLOSSARY OF TERMS

Matching

Match the key terms with their definitions.

KEY TERMS

1. _____ angioplasty

2. _____ atherectomy

3. _____ dissection

4. _____ hyperplasia

5. _____ stent

DEFINITION

a. A tear along the inner layer of an artery that results in the splitting or separation of the walls of a blood vessel

b. A tube-like structure placed inside a blood vessel to provide patency and support

c. A nonsurgical procedure to remove plaque from an artery using a special catheter with a device at the tip that cuts away the plaque

d. An abnormal increase in the number of cells; an increase in the number of smooth muscle cells within the intima in response to vessel injury

e. A surgical repair of a blood vessel by reconstructing or replacing part of the vessel. The procedure can be done with a balloon-tipped catheter that is used to enlarge a narrowing (stenosis) in a blood vessel

CHAPTER REVIEW

Multiple Choice

Complete each question by circling the best answer.

1. What is the primary consideration when deciding on the type of intervention for patients with arterial occlusive disease of the upper or lower extremities?
   a. location and extent of disease
   b. comorbid risk factors
   c. etiology of disease
   d. risk–benefit ratio of the procedure

2. Which of the following is NOT one of the endovascular treatments of choice for more extensive arterial stenosis?
   a. balloon angioplasty
   b. subintimal angioplasty
   c. mechanical atherectomy
   d. stent graft angioplasty

3. What are the main factors the Trans-Atlantic Inter-Society Consensus (TASC) II criteria uses to classify lesion severity?
   a. the type of lesions
   b. the etiology and severity of the disease
   c. the extension and etiology of the disease
   d. the location and anatomy of the disease

4. Which TASC II lesions are most appropriate to undergo endovascular intervention?
   a. TASC A and B lesions
   b. TASC C and D lesions
   c. TASC A and C lesions
   d. TASC B and D lesions

5. Which of the following is NOT associated with poor outcomes (high risk of failure) of endovascular procedures?
   a. diabetes
   b. renal failure
   c. coronary disease
   d. tibial disease

6. Which of the following is NOT a symptom of poor limb reperfusion after endovascular procedure?
   a. claudication
   b. restenosis
   c. rest pain
   d. ulcers

7. Why is relying on the patient's history to assess successful reperfusion of a limb often challenging?
   a. Patients are often active and work through symptoms.
   b. Patients are often sedentary and do not walk enough to produce symptoms.
   c. Patients are often diabetic and have significant nerve damage.
   d. Patients are often obese and cannot be sufficiently evaluated with duplex.

8. In a patient with claudication, by how much should an ABI increase to demonstrate significant improvement in limb perfusion?
   a. 0.10
   b. 0.15
   c. 0.20
   d. 0.95

9. When would duplex assessment of an angioplasty site NOT be indicated?
   a. calcified tibial arteries with an asymptomatic patient
   b. asymptomatic patient with monophasic tibial artery waveforms
   c. normal ABI with monophasic tibial artery waveforms
   d. normal ABI with triphasic tibial artery waveforms

10. Which of the following should be performed common femoral artery waveform is monophasic or has an abnormal acceleration time?
    a. assessment of the popliteal artery
    b. assessment of the profunda femoris artery
    c. assessment of the iliac arteries
    d. no additional assessments need to be made

11. If areas of lumen reduction or disturbed flow are identified by color Doppler, how should they next be assessed?
    a. power Doppler
    b. PW spectral Doppler
    c. B-mode
    d. angiography

12. When evaluating a prosthetic bypass graft or stent-graft, what velocity has been associated with graft thrombosis?

    a. <50 cm/s

    b. <75 cm/s

    c. <100 cm/s

    d. >180 cm/s

13. Which of the following is NOT part of the referral documentation for exams in the vascular lab following an endovascular procedure?

    a. indications for the referral

    b. type of intervention performed

    c. location of the intervention performed

    d. risk factors for underlying disease

14. With which of the following is the prevalence of restenosis after endovascular procedure in the femoropopliteal segment of the arterial tree highest?

    a. balloon angioplasty

    b. stent graft

    c. atherectomy

    d. angioplasty

15. What are the primary measurements used to classify stenosis severity at an interventional site?

    a. PSV and EDV

    b. EDV and Vr

    c. Vr only

    d. PSV and Vr

16. Several studies have shown a good correlation between stenosis of 70% or more at the site of previous endovascular procedures. What are the results?

    a. PSV >300 cm/s and Vr >2

    b. PSV >180 cm/s and Vr >2

    c. PSV >300 cm/s and Vr >3.5

    d. PSV >30 cm/s and Vr <2

17. Why are flow velocities in a stent (without evidence of restenosis) usually increased compared to velocities in a native artery?

    a. A stent decreases the compliance of the arterial wall.

    b. A stent increases the compliance of the arterial wall.

    c. A stent decreases the resistance of the tissue.

    d. A stent increases the resistance of the tissue.

18. A patient presents to the vascular lab for follow-up of a superficial femoral artery stent. Upon duplex assessment of the stented area, the stent walls were noted to be sharply angled in the vessel lumen. Turbulence on color was noted in the area. What do these findings suggest?

    a. in-stent stenosis

    b. stent deformation or kinking

    c. normally deployed stent

    d. myointimal hyperplasia development

19. During what period is endovascular intervention failure the highest?

    a. within first 6 months

    b. within first 12 months

    c. within first 18 months

    d. within first 24 months

20. When would abbreviated testing intervals for follow-up of an interventional site be appropriate?

    a. Following treatment of TASC A and B lesions.

    b. In patients with normal ABI duplex findings on initial surveillance.

    c. Following treatment of TASC C and D lesions.

    d. In patients treated with balloon angioplasty only.

Fill-in-the-Blank

1. The most common endovascular procedure to address an arterial stenosis is _____.

2. Focal endovascular interventions may not restore peripheral pulse because atherosclerosis is usually _____.

3. It has been estimated that approximately _____ of lesions treated with endovascular procedures will require another intervention within the first year.

4. Angioplasty of the _____ arteries is associated with a higher patency rate than for superficial femoral or popliteal artery angioplasty.

5. Follow-up or sequential duplex ultrasound exams are recommended after an endovascular procedure because atherosclerotic lesions often _____.

6. When performing surveillance after intervention, limb perfusion is evaluated by _____ testing and duplex scanning of angioplasty site.

7. A toe pressure of at least _____ is a good predictor of adequate perfusion to heal an ulcer.

8. The popliteal artery, tibioperoneal trunk, and peroneal arteries can be imaged with the patient in a _____ or lateral _____ position.

9. Toe pressure below 30 mm Hg is usually synonymous with _____.

10. In order to identify the highest peak systolic velocity in an area of abnormality, it is valuable to _____ the sample volume through the area.

11. The most common cause for restenosis independently of the endovascular procedure performed is _____.

12. When compared to angiography, duplex ultrasound of an interventional site provides hemodynamic information that gives a more precise assessment of _____ patency.

13. The functional significance of a stenosis should always be assessed with _____ testing.

14. Duplex ultrasound detection of a >50% stenosis proximal to, within, or distal to the endovascular intervention is interpreted as a(n) _____ finding.

15. A velocity ratio greater than 2 with associated lumen reduction, disturbed flow on color Doppler, and a focal velocity increase >180 cm/s all suggest a _____.

16. Classification of angioplasty site disease is commonly reported in one of three categories: <50% stenosis, _____ stenosis, and _____.

17. Peak systolic velocity values for grading in-stent stenosis are _____ than they are for atherosclerotic lesions in native vessels.

18. If damped, low-velocity waveforms are demonstrated in vessels distal to an angioplasty site, _____ of the angioplasty site is suggested.

19. Stent fracture, deformation, or kinking are abnormal findings that are associated with stent _____.

20. The outcome status following an additional intervention to restore patency following endovascular procedure is referred to as _____.

Short Answer

1. What are the two main reasons for vascular laboratory follow-up of interventional procedures?

2. Why is duplex ultrasound the diagnostic modality of choice for follow-up of patients with interventional procedures?

3. How should B-mode and color Doppler imaging be used when evaluating an interventional site?

4. When providing an interpretation of limb pressures and duplex ultrasound findings following endovascular intervention, what should the interpretive report include?

5. What is a typical surveillance schedule following endovascular intervention in a patient being treated for critical limb ischemia?

IMAGE EVALUATION/PATHOLOGY

Review the images and answer the following questions.

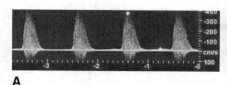
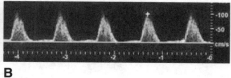
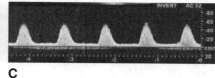

A B C

1. Which Doppler spectrum is most likely to be taken proximal to a stenosis?

2. Which Doppler spectrum is most likely to be taken at a stenosis?

3. Which Doppler spectrum is most likely to be taken distal to a stenosis?

4. The velocities seen on Doppler spectrum are consistent with what?

CASE STUDY

1. A 63-year-old female treated for a focal external iliac artery lesion with balloon angioplasty and stenting presents for a 6-month follow-up in the vascular lab. On assessing the stented area, you keep in mind that in this period, what would the most likely "failure" involve? On duplex ultrasound examination, you find PSV within the stented area of 150 cm/s and a PSV ratio of 1.8. What would you conclude? The patient describes symptoms of calf claudication, and the ABI reveals a drop of 0.2 (at rest) from the preprocedure value. What would you conclude from this additional information?

Special Considerations in Evaluating Nonatherosclerotic Arterial Pathology

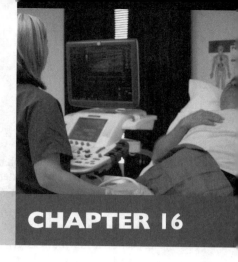

CHAPTER 16

REVIEW OF GLOSSARY OF TERMS

Matching

Match the key terms with their definitions.

KEY TERMS

1. _____ vascular arteritis

2. _____ giant cell arteritis

3. _____ Buerger's disease

4. _____ Takayasu's arteritis

5. _____ embolism

6. _____ aneurysm

7. _____ pseudoaneurysm

8. _____ arteriovenous fistula

DEFINITION

a. An obstruction or occlusion of a blood vessel by a transported clot of blood, mass, bacteria, or other foreign substance

b. An inflammatory disease that affects the blood vessels

c. A type of vascular arteritis that affects the aortic arch and its large branches

d. A type of vascular arteritis also known as thromboangiitis obliterans; it affects small- and medium-sized arteries

e. A type of vascular arteritis also known as temporal arteritis, which is associated with the superficial temporal artery and other arteries of the head and neck

f. An abnormal communication between an artery and a vein, which can be the result of iatrogenic injury or trauma or may be congenitally acquired

g. A dilation of an artery wall involving all three layers of the vessel wall

h. An expanding hematoma; a hole in the arterial wall that allows blood to leave the vessel and collect in the surrounding tissue

CHAPTER REVIEW

Multiple Choice

Complete each question by circling the best answer.

1. When using spectral Doppler, peak systolic velocities are routinely recorded. Under which conditions is it particularly useful to record end-diastolic velocities?
   a. Distal to a stenosis.
   b. When an aneurysm is present.
   c. When abnormally high- or low-resistance flow patterns are present.
   d. End-diastolic velocities should always be recorded.

2. Which layer of the vessel wall is most likely to undergo infiltration of white blood cells during the inflammatory process encountered with most arteritis diseases?
   a. the media layer
   b. the intima layer
   c. the adventitia layer
   d. both the intima and media equally

3. In a patient presenting with signs and symptoms of giant cell arteritis and asymmetric blood pressures, what should also be assessed?
   a. the aortic arch
   b. the lower extremity arteries
   c. the upper extremity arteries
   d. the digits

4. When assessing giant cell arteritis on grayscale imaging, an anechoic area is often present surrounding the affected vessel. How is this appearance often described on the image?
   a. doughnut
   b. halo
   c. macaroni
   d. burger

5. Which vessels are most commonly affected by Takayasu's arteritis?
   a. the common carotid arteries
   b. the innominate artery
   c. the axillary arteries
   d. the subclavian arteries

6. When present, where will lower extremity claudication symptoms with thromboangiitis obliterans most likely be localized?
   a. the arch of the foot
   b. the ankle
   c. the calf
   d. the thigh

7. What is an essential evaluation to determine a proper diagnosis of Buerger's disease?
   a. ankle or wrist arteries with spectral and color Doppler
   b. proximal large arteries with duplex ultrasound
   c. indirect testing of the calf with PVR waveforms
   d. digital evaluation with PPG waveforms

8. Which symptom would be typical in a patient with an arterial lesion due to radiation-induced arteritis?
   a. onset of claudication several months after completion of radiation treatment
   b. visual disturbances and jaw claudication
   c. ischemic ulcers of the digits during radiation treatment
   d. pulsatile mass in the area of radiation treatment

9. A cardiac source of arterial embolism can be seen with all the following EXCEPT:
   a. atrial fibrillation.
   b. endocarditis.
   c. mitral valve prolapse.
   d. left ventricle thrombus.

10. What term describes arterial embolization as a result of deep vein thrombosis in the presence of an intracardiac right to left shunt?
    a. cardioembolic disease
    b. Buerger's disease
    c. ventricular embolization
    d. paradoxic embolization

11. Pseudoaneurysms can be seen with all of the following EXCEPT:
    a. postcardiac catheterization.
    b. as an inflammatory response.
    c. at site of infection of synthetic grafts.
    d. with dialysis access grafts.

12. What does the "Yin-Yang" symbol describe?
    a. the flow pattern in an arteriovenous fistula
    b. the flow pattern in an aneurysm sac
    c. the flow pattern at an area of dissection
    d. the flow pattern in a pseudoaneurysm sac

13. What are most iatrogenic arteriovenous fistula the result of?
    a. femoral artery catheterization
    b. central venous line placement
    c. penetrating wounds
    d. total knee replacement

14. Which statement about popliteal artery entrapment syndrome is FALSE?
    a. It affects males more frequently than females.
    b. It often affects both limbs.
    c. It is an acquired condition.
    d. It is a congenital condition.

15. What is the preferred maneuver to diagnose popliteal artery entrapment syndrome?
    a. ABI with treadmill exercise testing
    b. duplex assessment with active plantar flexion
    c. duplex assessment involving rotating the limb
    d. physiologic testing with limb dependent then elevated

16. Which condition is a congenital disorder of connective tissue often resulting in aneurysm formation?
    a. Buerger's disease
    b. Takayasu's disease
    c. Ehlers–Danlos syndrome
    d. Kawasaki syndrome

17. What is the primary site for aneurysm development associated with Marfan's syndrome?
    a. the abdominal aorta
    b. the common femoral artery
    c. the popliteal artery
    d. the aortic arch

18. What is a devastating complication of Ehlers–Danlos syndrome?
    a. aneurysm
    b. arterial rupture
    c. thrombosis
    d. atherosclerosis

19. An 80-year-old female presents to the vascular lab with a palpable thrill in the right groin after catheterization procedure. Upon duplex assessment of the area, increased diastolic flow is noted in the very proximal right common femoral artery, and prominent pulsatility is noted in right common femoral vein. A significant color bruit is noted in the area as well. What do these findings suggest?
    a. arteriovenous fistula of the common femoral vessels
    b. acute arterial embolization
    c. right common femoral artery dissection
    d. pseudoaneurysm of the right common femoral artery

20. A 42-year-old male smoker presents to the vascular lab with ischemic digit ulcers, on his fingers as well as his toes. The patient also notes some tingling in his feet. What should be suspected in this patient?
    a. thromboangiitis obliterans
    b. popliteal artery entrapment
    c. Takayasu's arteritis
    d. aneurysmal disease of the subclavian artery

21. A 66-year-old female presents to the vascular lab with sudden onset of severe right lower extremity pain, pallor, and pulselessness. The patient describes a history of atrial fibrillation. What should be suspected in this patient?
    a. right common femoral artery pseudoaneurysm
    b. radiation-induced arteritis in the iliac system
    c. cardiac source acute embolization to the right leg
    d. acute thrombosis of a popliteal artery aneurysm

22. A 73-year-old female presents to the vascular lab with temporal headaches, jaw claudication, visual disturbances, and a palpable cord over her forehead. What should be suspected in this patient?
    a. thromboangiitis obliterans
    b. giant cell arteritis
    c. Takayasu's arteritis
    d. pseudoaneurysm of the temporal artery

23. A 53-year-old male presents to the vascular lab with a pulsatile mass in his right groin. The patient recently underwent a cardiac catheterization procedure. Upon duplex evaluation, an encapsulated mass is noted with to-and-fro flow noted in a channel connecting the right common femoral artery to the mass. What do these findings most likely represent?
    a. arteriovenous fistula of the common femoral vessels
    b. acute arterial occlusion
    c. right common femoral artery dissection
    d. pseudoaneurysm of the right common femoral artery

24. A 32-year-old Asian female presents to the vascular lab with weak radial pulses and several transient ischemic attacks. What should be suspected in this patient?
    a. thromboangiitis obliterans
    b. giant cell arteritis
    c. atherosclerotic disease of the carotid arteries
    d. Takayasu's arteritis

25. A 75-year-old male presents to the vascular lab with cool, pulseless limb shortly after catheterization through the right common femoral artery. Upon duplex assessment, echogenic material was noted in the common femoral artery with a staccato type waveform obtained just proximal to this area. What do these findings suggest?

a. arteriovenous fistula of the common femoral vessels
b. right common femoral artery dissection
c. acute arterial occlusion of the right common femoral artery
d. pseudoaneurysm of the right common femoral artery

Fill-in-the-Blank

1. The etiology of arteritis is unknown; however, the inflammatory process often involves a(n) _____ condition.

2. The symptoms described by patients suffering from some forms of arteritis are often _____ to the symptoms of patients with atherosclerosis.

3. The form of arteritis that is rarely seen in patients younger than 50 years is _____.

4. On a B-mode imaging in a patient with Takayasu's arteritis, circumferential thickening of the vessel wall is often noted and has been termed the _____ sign.

5. Takayasu's disease process, along with the possible occlusion of the vessel lumen, may be complicated by the formation of _____.

6. While giant cell and Takayasu's arteritis are more common in _____; thromboangiitis obliterans is more common in _____.

7. Although smoking is always present in the history of patients suffering from Buerger's disease, it is even more prominent in areas where smoking involves _____.

8. Although radiation-induced arteritis lesions often resemble atherosclerotic lesions, radiation-induced lesions are usually _____ and _____ in nature, whereas atherosclerotic lesions, although focal, tend to be more widespread.

9. In a patient with abrupt onset of leg pain, the absence of plaque and collateral flow most likely indicates _____ as the cause of symptoms.

10. It has been shown that 80% to 99% of arterial embolisms have a _____ source.

11. Epidemiologic studies have shown that the site outside the cerebral circulation that is most commonly affected by arterial embolization is the _____.

12. The most common site of iatrogenic pseudoaneurysm is the _____.

13. The characteristic flow pattern observed on a Doppler spectrum at the level of the neck of a pseudoaneurysm is often referred to as _____.

14. A bruit is found on _____, whereas a thrill is found on _____.

15. Arterial closure devices used postcatheterization have occasionally been the cause of _____.

16. Popliteal artery entrapment occurs when the popliteal artery is compressed by the medial head of the _____ muscle.

17. Popliteal artery entrapment is suspected when a young patient with no risk factors for atherosclerosis presents with _____.

18. While Takayasu's arteritis frequently causes stenosis of the aortic arch arteries, the formation of aneurysm associated with this disorder are the more frequent _____ complication.

19. Behcet's syndrome has been associated as a source of non-atherosclerotic _____.

20. An aneurysm can be diagnosed when the diameter of a vessel is increased by _____ compared to an adjacent proximal vessel.

Short Answer

1. Why can nonatherosclerotic diseases usually be recognized and assessed clinically?

2. What differences are noted on the B-mode, grayscale image between the vessels affected by atherosclerosis versus those affected by arteritis?

3. What differences in flow patterns can be seen between pseudoaneurysms and arteriovenous fistulae?

IMAGE EVALUATION/PATHOLOGY

Review the images and answer the following questions.

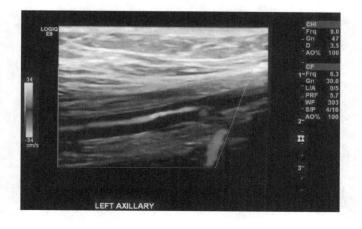

1. What does the appearance of the lumen and the location of the disease in this image suggest?

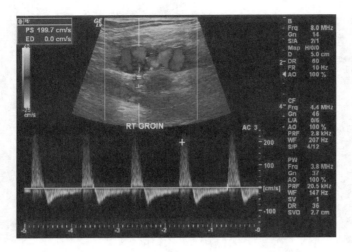

2. What does this Doppler spectrum show and where does it commonly occur?

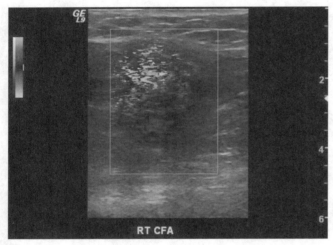

A

3. What is demonstrated in these images?

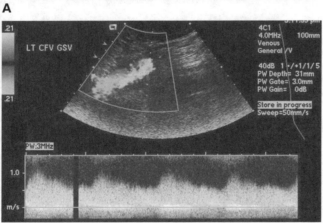

B

CASE STUDY

1. A female patient presents to the vascular lab with a 30 mm Hg brachial blood pressure difference between the right and left arm. The patient has no known risk factors for atherosclerotic disease. What conditions would you consider in this patient? What additional history questions would you ask in order to help determine the disease process in this patient?

   Upon duplex assessment, the subclavian and axillary arteries appear to have concentric wall thickening, consistent with the "macaroni" sign, with increased peak systolic velocities. What condition would these findings be consistent with?

2. A 19-year-old male presents to the vascular lab with claudication symptoms at the calf level bilaterally. He notices the calf pain with walking but not with running. He does not have any other relevant risk factors or relevant medical history. Based on his age, symptoms, and history, your first instinct would lead you to focus on which area? Upon examination of the area of focus, you cannot find anything remarkable (no increased velocities), but the spatial relation of the artery and vein does not seem "quite right." What probable cause for his pain do you start thinking of? To confirm your diagnosis, you decide to obtain Doppler spectrum and velocities in the artery with duplex ultrasound while the patient performs which maneuver?

3. A 67-year-old male patient presents to the vascular lab after an interventional catheterization procedure with access through the right brachial artery. What conditions would you consider could be present in this patient?

   Upon physical examination, the right radial artery pulse is weak, and no bruit is heard in the area of the access site. Duplex assessment reveals echogenic material with in the lumen of the brachial artery with staccato-like waveforms noted in the proximal subclavian artery. What do these findings suggest?

PART FIVE

PERIPHERAL VENOUS

Duplex Ultrasound Imaging of the Lower Extremity Venous System

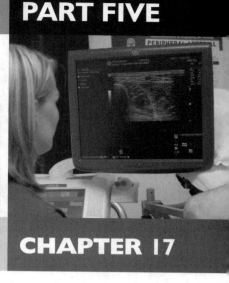

REVIEW OF GLOSSARY OF TERMS

Matching

Match the key terms with their definitions.

KEY TERMS

1. _b_ deep vein

2. _f_ superficial vein

3. _d_ perforating vein

4. _a_ acute thrombus

5. _e_ chronic thrombus

6. _c_ valve

DEFINITION

a. Newly formed clotted blood within a vein, generally less than 14 days old
b. A vein that is the companion vessel to an artery and travels within the deep muscular compartments of the leg
c. An inward projection of the intimal layer of a vein wall producing two semilunar leaflets, which present the retrograde movement of blood flow
d. A small vein that connects the deep and superficial venous systems; a vein that passes between the deep and superficial compartments of the leg
e. Clotted blood within a vein that has generally been present for a period of several weeks or months
f. A vein that is superior to the muscular compartments of the leg; travels within superficial fascial compartments; has no corresponding companion artery

ANATOMY AND PHYSIOLOGY REVIEW

Image Labeling

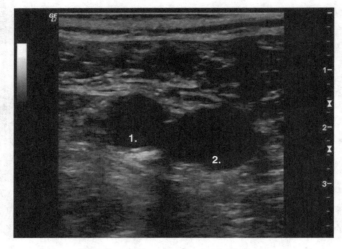

1 CFA
2 CFV

1. A transverse view at the level of the groin.

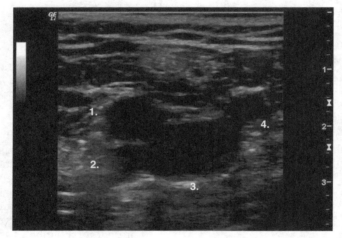

1 SFA
2 PFA
3 CFV
4 GSV

2. A transverse view at the level of the groin.

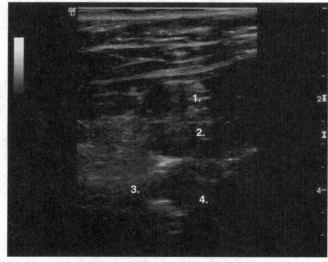

1 SFA
2 FV
3 DFA
4 DFV

3. A transverse view through the proximal thigh.

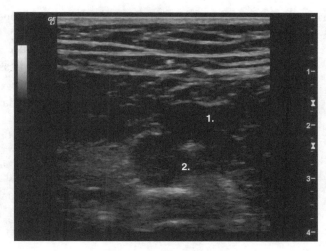

4. A transverse view through the mid-thigh.

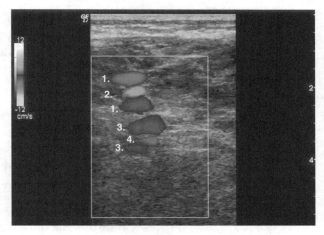

5. A transverse view through mid-calf.

CHAPTER REVIEW

Multiple Choice

Complete each question by circling the best answer.

1. Which category of veins are the main conduit for blood, are surrounded by muscle, and have an accompanying artery?
   a. deep veins
   b. superficial veins
   c. muscular veins
   d. perforators

2. What is the main function of the superficial venous system under normal conditions?
   a. To provide a collateral pathway for the deep veins.
   b. To connect with the deep system through perforating veins.
   c. To help regulate the body temperature.
   d. To provide a reservoir for blood.

3. In which way do valves in perforating veins ensure that blood moves, under normal conditions?
   a. dissipate around the perforator
   b. from the superficial to the deep system
   c. from the deep to the superficial system
   d. stay in the superficial system

4. From epidemiologic studies, what percentage of patients develop postthrombotic symptoms?
   a. 10%
   b. 30%
   c. 50%
   d. 90%

5. Which limb of Virchow's triad is demonstrated by a venous thrombus that starts at a valve cusp?

    a. wall injury

    b. hypercoagulability

    c. stasis

    d. congenital component

6. A patient presents to the vascular lab for lower extremity venous evaluation. The patient has known Factor V Leiden genetic factor. Under what risk factor of Virchow's triad does this patient fall?

    a. wall injury

    b. hypercoagulability

    c. stasis

    d. congenital component

7. Many patients with venous thrombosis are asymptomatic; however, when symptoms occur, what are some of the most common?

    a. extremity pain, tenderness, and swelling

    b. muscle pain with exercise

    c. ulcerations on toes and thickened toenails

    d. extremity weakness, numbness, and tingling

8. What would a high probability for DVT correspond to on Well's score?

    a. <3 points

    b. >2 point

    c. >3 points

    d. >5 points

9. When can a false-negative D-dimer be seen in the presence of DVT?

    a. The patient has underlying malignancy.

    b. The patient has active inflammation/infection.

    c. Assay cannot detect high level of fibrin.

    d. Assay cannot detect low levels of fibrin.

10. For routine operation of a vascular lab, the use of a high-frequency linear transducer (10 to 18 MHz) is recommended for the evaluation of which of the following?

    a. superficial vein reflux

    b. perforators

    c. distal femoral vein

    d. iliac veins

11. Why will using a reverse Trendelenburg position to examine the lower extremity venous system make the exam more difficult?

    a. Veins will be collapsed.

    b. Veins will be under low pressure.

    c. Veins will be deeper.

    d. Veins without thrombus will be harder to compress.

12. What is the primary method used to determine the presence of thrombus in the extremity veins?

    a. color-flow Doppler

    b. transducer compression of the veins

    c. spectral Doppler waveforms

    d. sagittal B-mode images

13. Which of the following is NOT a normal qualitative Doppler feature evaluated in the lower extremity venous system?

    a. continuity of signal

    b. spontaneity of signal

    c. phasicity of signal

    d. augmentation of signal

14. Which of the following large deep veins are commonly bifid?

    a. the profunda and popliteal veins

    b. the femoral and popliteal veins

    c. the external iliac and femoral veins

    d. the common femoral and popliteal veins

15. Which vessels are NOT routinely evaluated in a lower extremity venous duplex examination?

    a. femoral vein

    b. great saphenous vein

    c. anterior tibial veins

    d. small saphenous vein

16. Which veins are one of the major blood reservoirs located in the calf?

    a. the tibial veins

    b. the small saphenous vein

    c. the soleal veins

    d. the popliteal vein

17. What do bright intraluminal echoes and well-attached thrombus suggest?

    a. acute thrombosis

    b. chronic thrombosis

    c. too much gain

    d. risks of embolization

18. In what case will indirect assessment of the iliac veins and IVC using Doppler at the common femoral veins suggest evidence of obstruction?

    a. The Doppler spectrum exhibits phasicity.

    b. The Doppler spectrum exhibits pulsatility.

    c. The Doppler spectrum exhibits continuity.

    d. The Doppler spectrum ceases with Valsalva.

19. During a lower extremity venous duplex examination, a thin, white structure is noticed moving freely in the lumen of the vein. What does this most likely represent?
    a. valve leaflet
    b. mobile thrombus
    c. dissection
    d. chronic scarring

20. Which of the following is a normal response to venous flow with a Valsalva maneuver?
    a. augmented flow
    b. phasicity of flow
    c. continuous flow
    d. cessation of flow

21. A patient presents to the vascular lab with sudden onset of left lower extremity pain and swelling. Upon duplex examination, lightly echogenic material is noted within a dilated femoral vein, and the femoral vein does not compress with applied transducer pressure. What do these findings suggest?
    a. chronic deep venous thrombosis
    b. acute deep venous thrombosis
    c. acute superficial venous thrombosis
    d. superficial venous valvular incompetence

22. When a patient presents with right heart failure, what impact is often observed in the spectral Doppler waveform in the lower extremities?
    a. increased pulsatility
    b. continuous flow
    c. decreased phasicity
    d. loss of augmentation

23. A patient presents to the emergency department with a massively swollen right lower extremity which is extremely painful and bluish in color. What do these findings suggest?
    a. May–Thurner syndrome
    b. phlegmasia alba dolens
    c. phlegmasia cerulen dolens
    d. venous gangrene

24. Which treatment option is typically reserved for emergent situations in larger veins of the iliofemoral region?
    a. heparin
    b. coumadin
    c. elastic stockings
    d. thrombolysis

25. What is the primary treatment of acute lower extremity deep venous thrombosis?
    a. thrombolysis
    b. anticoagulation
    c. thrombectomy
    d. elastic stockings

Fill-in-the-Blank

1. Duplex ultrasound for the evaluation of the deep and superficial venous system has largely replaced _venography_ for the detection of DVT.

2. Duplex ultrasound has the capability to diagnose, localize, and determine the age of _thrombus_.

3. The primary mechanism for the formation of venous thrombosis which includes venous stasis, vessel wall injury, and a hypercoagulable state is known as _Virchow's triad_

4. The fact that DVT is often undiagnosed or underdiagnosed is likely because DVT is frequently _____.

5. The development of venous thrombosis is determined by a balance between clotting factors and _coagulation inhibitors_

6. Tachypnea, tachycardia, and chest pain are often signs of _PE_.

7. A palpable cord along the medial aspect of the lower extremity would be a clinical sign for _VTE_.

8. A patient with localized tenderness with limb swelling and a recent history of major surgery would score ____3____ points based on Well's scoring of risk factors.

9. The clinical diagnosis of DVT has ___poor___ sensitivity and specificity.

10. Appropriate positioning of the patient for a lower extremity venous evaluation includes having the patient lie on their back with their knee slightly bent and the hip _slightly externally_ rotated.

11. The evaluation of the IVC and iliac veins in most adult patients would require the use of a ___2.5 MHz___ transducer.

12. The position described as the tilting of the exam table during a venous exam so that the legs are approximately 20 degrees lower than the upper body is called _reversed Trendelenburg_.

13. Transducer compression of the extremity veins should NOT be performed in a _longitudinal_ plane as it is easy to roll off the veins from this approach.

14. The junction of the great saphenous vein with the common femoral vein usually occurs _superiorly_ to the bifurcation of the superficial and deep femoral arteries.

15. The main venous outflow for the calf is the _popliteal vein_.

16. The extension of the small saphenous vein above the popliteal fossa is referred to as the vein of _Giacomini_, or currently the _cranial_ extension of the small saphenous vein.

17. It is not unusual for the _small saphenous_ vein to share a common trunk with the gastrocnemius vein.

18. The posterior tibial and peroneal veins typically communicate with the _soleal_ veins.

19. The only way to adequately image the content of the venous lumen to exclude DVT when performing compression is to view the vessel in _transverse_.

20. The process of a thrombus continuing to shrink and fill less of the vein can be known as _recanalization_.

21. When using Doppler, if there is thrombosis between the level of the transducer and the site of distal compression, the result will be _____ with the compression.

22. Unilateral pulsatile venous flow can be associated with _arteriovenous fistulae_.

23. Compression of the left common iliac vein by the right common iliac artery can result in _May-Thurner_ syndrome.

24. A nonvascular, anechoic, well-defined, oval mass found incidentally during a lower extremity venous duplex evaluation most likely represents a(n) _acute thrombus_.

25. Computed tomography venography and magnetic resonance venography are often used to evaluate the status of the _iliac_ veins.

Short Answer

1. What three things are the examiner trying to assess when performing a venous duplex examination?

the presence or absence of thrombus.
The relative risk of the thrombus dislodging & traveling to the lungs
The competence of the contained valves

2. Why is a pulmonary embolism more likely to occur from the deep venous system versus the superficial venous system?

The squeezing action in the deep veins can be the mechanism for dislodging a contained thrombus.

3. Why is a thrombus in the anterior tibial veins rare?

Because they do not communicate with the prime source of thrombi in the leg - the soleal sinus veins

4. What are some situations that may lead to false-positive results during the compression portion of an extremity venous evaluation?

body habitus
femoral vein that passes through the adductor canal

5. What are the advantages and disadvantages of the new oral anticoagulants?

advantages: no dietary restrictions, no monitoring
disadvantages: have shorter half-lives, no antidote

IMAGE EVALUATION/PATHOLOGY

Review the images and answer the following questions.

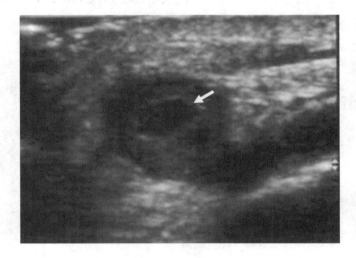

1. What is the arrow pointing at?

extremely acute thrombus

2. What does the circumferential area just inside the vessel wall represent?

fibrin net

3. What was the technique/tool used to allow for visualization in this image?

Transverse view with increased gain

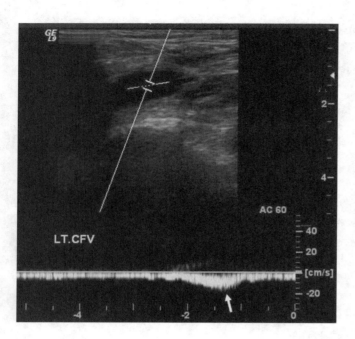

4. What would create this waveform in the common femoral vein?

an abnormal continuous pattern

Flow that lacks respiratory phasicity

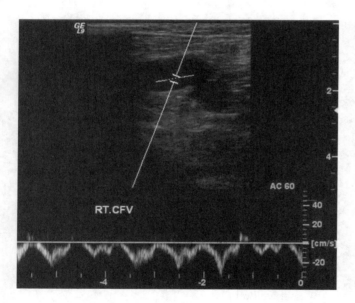

5. What would create this waveform in the common femoral vein?

an abnormal pulsatile

Flow that is spontaneous and augments with distal compression but appears pulsatile

CASE STUDY

1. An 86-year-old male presents in the vascular laboratory with a history of right leg pitting edema for 1 week. The right leg is red and warm from midthigh to the ankle. The patient has prostate cancer and IVC filter placement because of previous DVT.

   DVT in the right lower ext...

   a. What is your first impression?

   DVT in the right lower extremity

   b. Calculate the Well's score for this patient.

   3

   c. On duplex examination, you find a continuous Doppler spectrum at the right and left common femoral veins. Do you revise your first impression?

   Bilateral CFV continuous Doppler spectra
   yes

   d. What should you focus on next, given the patient history, and what do you expect to find?

   explore the IVC

2. A 32-year-old female presents in the vascular lab with a history of pain for 3 weeks in the upper to mid-calf on the right leg. She is healthy, athletic, of normal weight, and does not use birth control pills.

   a. Calculate the Well's score for this patient.

   -1

   b. The protocol for your lab does not routinely include the evaluation of veins below the knee. Is this a case when an exception is warranted? Why?

   c. On examination, you find DVT in the peroneal veins. The referring physician orders serial exams, and the thrombus appears to propagate toward the popliteal vein. What could explain the development and progression of DVT in this patient?

Duplex Ultrasound Imaging of the Upper Extremity Venous System

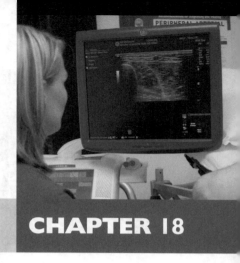

REVIEW OF GLOSSARY OF TERMS

Matching

Match the key terms with their definitions.

KEY TERMS

1. __C__ valve

2. __D__ superficial vein

3. __E__ chronic thrombus

4. __A__ deep vein

5. __B__ acute thrombus

DEFINITION

a. A vein that is the companion vessel to an artery and travels within the deep muscular compartments of the leg or arm

b. Newly formed clotted blood within a vein, generally less than 14 days old

c. An inward projection of the intimal layer of a vein wall producing two semilunar leaflets that prevent the retrograde movement of blood flow

d. A vein that is superior to the muscular compartments of the leg or arm; travels within the superficial fascial compartments and has no corresponding companion artery

e. Clotted blood within a vein that has generally been present for a period of several weeks or months

ANATOMY AND PHYSIOLOGY REVIEW

Image Labeling

1. IJV
2. CCA

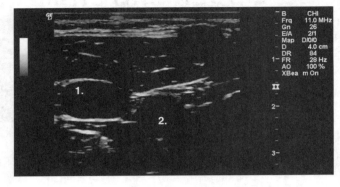

1. Transverse image through the mid-neck.

1. cephalic v
2. SCV

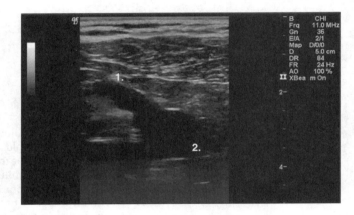

2. Transverse image of the proximal upper arm.

1. basilic vein
2 brachial vein
3 brachial artery

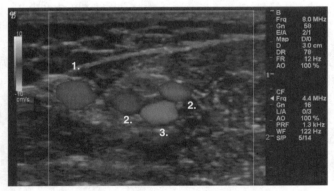

3. Transverse image of the mid-upper arm.

CHAPTER REVIEW

Multiple Choice

Complete each question by circling the best answer.

1. **What is the main reason that venous thrombosis in the upper extremities has become more common?**
   a. a more sedentary lifestyle
   b. increased injury to vein walls
   c. an increase in hypercoagulable disease states
   d. decreased rates of prophylactic anticoagulation

2. **Unlike the lower extremities, what do the upper extremities NOT have that may allow spontaneous thrombus formation?**
   a. deep veins
   b. superficial veins
   c. soleal sinuses
   d. respiratory phasic flow dynamics

3. **What is venous thrombosis secondary to compression of the subclavian vein at the thoracic inlet?**
   a. Paget–Schroetter syndrome
   b. May–Thurner syndrome
   c. Raynaud's syndrome
   d. phlegmasia

4. **A patient presents to the vascular lab for upper extremity venous evaluation with face swelling and prominent veins on the chest and neck. What do these findings suggest?**
   a. subclavian vein thrombosis
   b. cephalic vein thrombosis
   c. internal jugular vein thrombosis
   d. superior vena cava thrombosis

5. **Transducer compressions are limited over several veins in the upper extremity because of limited access from bony structures. What are the most common veins that are NOT able to be compressed?**
   a. brachiocephalic and subclavian veins
   b. subclavian and axillary veins
   c. cephalic and basilic veins
   d. brachial and radial veins

6. **What is the most appropriate transducer for mapping of the upper extremity superficial venous system?**
   a. 5 to 10 MHz straight linear array
   b. 5 to 10 MHz curved linear array
   c. 10 to 18 MHz straight linear array
   d. 3.5 to 5 MHz curved linear or sector array

7. **Why are the subclavian and jugular veins assessed with the patient lying flat?**
   a. To reduce hydrostatic pressure
   b. To reduce compression from the clavicle
   c. To reduce heart pulsatility
   d. To reduce respiration

8. **How does the external jugular vein lie in relation to the internal jugular vein?**
   a. anterior
   b. superior
   c. deep
   d. posterior

9. **With which vein does the brachial vein become the axillary vein at the confluence?**
   a. cephalic vein
   b. radial vein
   c. basilic vein
   d. median cubital vein

10. **During an upper extremity venous examination, the technologist has made the patient take in a quick, deep breath through pursed lips while viewing the subclavian vein. What is the purpose of this action?**
    a. Dilate the subclavian vein.
    b. Increase color filling of the vein.
    c. Collapse/coapt the subclavian vein.
    d. Show pulsatile flow in the vein.

11. **In the upper extremity, in general, which venous system is larger?**
    a. deep system
    b. superficial system
    c. deep and superficial of equal size
    d. perforating system

12. **During an upper extremity venous duplex examination, the technologist notes significant pulsatility in the spectral Doppler waveform from the internal jugular vein. What does this finding suggest?**
    a. proximal venous obstruction
    b. distal venous obstruction
    c. normal findings for the IJV
    d. superficial venous obstruction

13. Which vessel may NOT be routinely evaluated in a UE venous duplex examination but is often added in the event of significant thrombosis?

    a. internal jugular vein

    b. subclavian vein

    c. basilic vein

    d. external jugular vein

14. Because of the location of the brachiocephalic veins, documentation of patency of these vessels is usually performed with which of the following?

    a. Grayscale image with additional color-flow and spectral Doppler images

    b. Grayscale imaging alone

    c. Grayscale image with and without transducer compression

    d. Color-flow imaging alone

15. Which vessel connects the basilic and cephalic veins?

    a. radial veins

    b. anterior jugular vein

    c. medial cubital vein

    d. interosseous vein

16. Which forearm vessels are NOT routinely evaluated during upper extremity venous duplex testing?

    a. basilic and cephalic veins

    b. basilic and ulnar veins

    c. cephalic and radial veins

    d. radial and ulnar veins

17. A 34-year-old female presents to the vascular lab with a 1-day history of arm swelling and redness. The patient has recently had a PICC line inserted. During the duplex evaluation, the axillary and subclavian veins are incompressible with hypoechoic echoes noted within their lumens. What do these findings suggest?

    a. chronic venous thrombosis

    b. acute venous thrombosis

    c. acute venous insufficiency

    d. normal findings in these vessels

18. A 78-year-old male presents to the vascular lab with right arm swelling for the past several days. The patient notes that he is currently being treated for cancer. During the upper extremity duplex examination, decreased pulsatility is noted in the right internal jugular and subclavian veins as well as rouleaux (slow) flow formation. What do these findings suggest?

    a. normal upper extremity duplex examination

    b. a more distal obstruction, likely in the brachial and cephalic veins

    c. a more proximal obstruction, likely in the brachiocephalic vein or superior vena cava

    d. congestive heart failure

19. During an upper extremity venous duplex evaluation, color flow is noted filling the axillary vein. However, in a transverse view, the axillary vein is noted to be only partially compressible. Which of the following could explain these findings?

    a. Color priority set too low and color gain too high

    b. Color scale too high and color gain too low

    c. Color priority and scale too high

    d. Color packet size and gain too low

20. A 22-year-old male patient presents to the vascular lab with a 3-day history of left arm swelling with no apparent injury or risk factors. Upon further questioning, the patient does state that he has recently begun weight training. What do the vascular technologist suspect in this patient?

    a. effort thrombosis

    b. superficial venous thrombosis

    c. superior vena cava syndrome

    d. lymphedema

Fill-in-the-Blank

1. The _Superficial_ veins of the arm are more affected by venous thrombosis than in the legs.

2. Signs and symptoms of upper extremity venous thrombosis are _Similar_ to symptoms in the lower extremity.

3. Thrombosis in the upper extremity veins is now most commonly caused by more frequent introduction of _needles_ and _catheters_ into arm veins.

4. Common veins to use for catheter placement and, therefore, for venous thrombosis are the _subclavian_ vein and the _internal jugular_ vein.

5. Veins that are typically used for the insertion of a PICC line are the _basilic_ or the _cephalic_.

6. Individuals who present with upper extremity thrombosis secondary to compression of the subclavian vein at the thoracic inlet have what is termed _effort_ thrombosis or _Paget Schroetter_ syndrome.

7. Superior vena cava syndrome often causes facial _swelling_ and prominent, dilated _chest wall_ collateral veins.

8. _Asymptomatic_ patients may present for upper extremity venous evaluation prior to catheter placement, venous mapping for bypass, and before placement of pacemaker wires.

9. As in the lower extremities, gentle compression with the transducer is applied over upper extremity veins to cause the walls to _coapt or close_.

10. Compression of the _brachiocephalic_ and _subclavian_ veins is usually not performed because of the position of these vessels in relation to the bony structures of the shoulder.

11. To evaluate the internal jugular, brachiocephalic, subclavian, axillary, and brachial veins, a _5-10_ MHz transducer is typically used; however, it is helpful to use a _10-18_ MHz transducer when evaluating small forearm veins as well as superficial upper extremity veins.

12. When sitting up or lying with the head elevated, hydrostatic pressure causes the jugular and subclavian veins to _collapse_; therefore, it is preferable to evaluate these vessels with the patient lying _supine_.

13. Evaluation of the jugular veins should be included in the upper extremity evaluation because they can be involved in the _thrombotic_ process or can provide _collateral_ pathways in the presence of upper extremity thrombosis.

14. The typical landmark used to identify the internal jugular vein is the _common carotid_ artery.

15. Hypoechoic material visualized within the lumen on a noncompressible, dilated vein is consistent with _acute_ venous thrombosis.

16. Flow reversal in the internal or external jugular veins is often associated with ipsilateral _brachiocephalic_ vein thrombus.

17. The median cubital vein connects the cephalic and basilic veins and is commonly used for _venipuncture_.

18. In veins that are partially thrombosed, the spectral Doppler signal is typically _continuous_ in nature but should display augmentation with distal compression.

19. One method to help determine patency of the central veins is to compare the _symmetry_ of the signal from the right and left sides.

20. Spectral Doppler characteristics of the upper extremity venous system include respiratory _phasicity_ and pronounced _pulsatility_ in the more centrally located vessels.

Short Answer

1. Compare the spectral Doppler waveforms from the upper extremity veins and the lower extremity veins.

respiratory phasicity in both pronounced pulsatility in upper extremities, especially in the ones closer to the heart

2. What methods are used to assess the jugular and subclavian veins that cannot by compressed by the transducer?

grayscale, color, & spectral Doppler.

3. What conditions can cause nonpulsatile, continuous flow to be present in the upper extremity venous system.

nonpulsatile Continuous flow is caused by proximal obstruction, partial thrombosis & external compression

4. What alterations can be seen in the upper extremity venous Doppler signals in the presence of a hemodialysis fistula?

pulsatile flow w/ elevated velocities respiratory variations may not be present

IMAGE EVALUATION/PATHOLOGY

Review the images and answer the following questions.

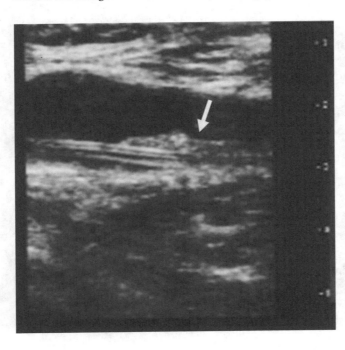

1. A 46-year-old female presents to the vascular lab for evaluation of catheter placement. The image was obtained during the duplex evaluation. Describe the findings in this image.

a thrombosis on a catheter

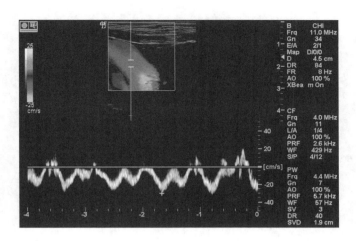

2. Describe the spectral Doppler waveform seen in the image. Which vessel is this likely taken from?

normal respiratory phasic flow
subclavian vein

CASE STUDY

1. A 75-year-old female presents to the vascular lab with right upper extremity swelling for the past 3 to 4 days. She has recently had a PICC line inserted through the cephalic vein. Upon duplex evaluation, the cephalic vein near the PICC line is incompressible and dilated with hypoechoic echoes present in the lumen. Additionally, the distal subclavian vein demonstrates hypoechoic echoes within its lumen and is Doppler silent.

   a. Assuming the brachial and basilic veins are patent, what would the spectral Doppler findings likely be in these vessels?

   a thrombosis in the subclavian + cephalic veins

   b. What other vessels would need to be evaluated in this patient? Given the history and the limited findings above, where else might be suspect for thrombus development? What are some treatment options for this patient?

   axillary, ijv, ejv, + brachiocephalic veins

2. A 19-year-old male presents to the vascular lab for suspected Paget–Schroetter syndrome. What symptoms and history would you expect this patient to have? Which vessel(s) would be most important to assess in this patient? Why?

   swelling athletic
   subclavian vein
   in Paget-Schroetter syndrome the subclavian vein is involved in thrombosis

Ultrasound Evaluation and Mapping of the Superficial Venous System

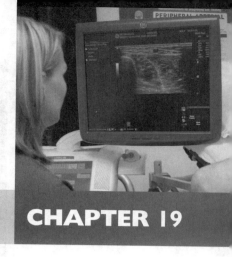

REVIEW OF GLOSSARY TERMS

Matching

Match the key terms with their definitions.

KEY TERMS

1. __C__ great saphenous vein

2. __E__ small saphenous vein

3. __B__ perforator vein

4. __F__ mapping

5. __D__ recanalization

6. __A__ varicosities

DEFINITION

a. Dilated, tortuous superficial veins

b. A vein that connects from the superficial venous system to the deep system

c. A superficial vein forming at the level of the medial malleolus; courses along medial calf and thigh

d. A vein that is now patent but had previously been thrombosed

e. A superficial vein that courses along the posterior aspect of the calf, terminating into the popliteal vein

f. Evaluating the patency, position, depth, and size of the superficial venous system for use as bypass conduit or other surgical procedures

ANATOMY AND PHYSIOLOGY REVIEW

Image Labeling

Complete the labels in the images that follow.

1 great saphenous v

2 Superficial fascia

3 muscular fascia

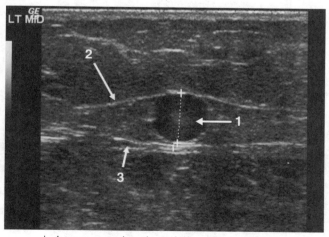

1. A transverse view through the mid-medial thigh.

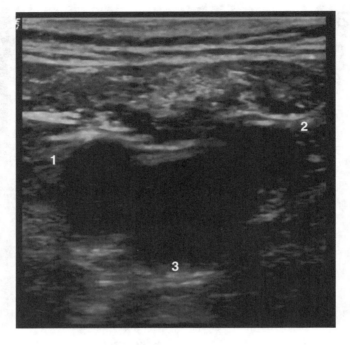

1 CFA
2 GSV
3 CFV

2. A transverse view at the saphenofemoral junction.

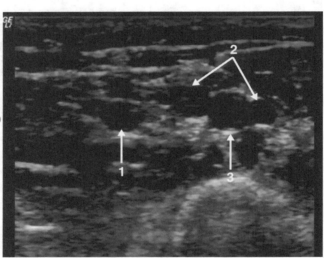

1. Basilic vein
2. Brachial vein
3. Brachial artery

3. A transverse view through the mid-upper arm.

CHAPTER REVIEW

Multiple Choice

Complete each question by circling the best answer.

1. Which of the following characteristics are assessed during preoperative evaluation of the superficial venous system?

    a. vein patency

    b. vein depth and size

    c. vein position

    d. all of the above

2. How many common configurations does the thigh portion of the great saphenous vein have?

    a. 10

    b. 2

    c. 4

    d. 5

3. What is a vein that penetrates the muscular fascia of the leg and connects the superficial system to the deep system?
   a. accessory saphenous vein
   b. perforating vein
   c. deep muscular vein
   d. venous sinus

4. To maximize venous pressure and distention, in what position should the patient's limbs be placed when mapping the superficial venous system?
   a. dependent
   b. elevated
   c. contracted
   d. adducted

5. What measures can be taken to ensure that a patient's vessels do not vasoconstrict?
   a. Keep the exam room cool and the patient uncovered.
   b. Keep the exam room cool but cover the patient, only exposing the limb being evaluated.
   c. Keep the exam room warm and cover the patient, only exposing the limb being evaluated.
   d. Keep the exam room warm and only cover the foot of the limb being evaluated.

6. Because superficial veins are under low pressure and just under the skin, what type of transducer compression must be used to compress these veins?
   a. light
   b. heavy
   c. moderate
   d. extreme

7. Which of the following describes the proper technique for marking a superficial vein in a longitudinal image orientation?
   a. Vein should appear ovoid in shape; transducer should be perpendicular to skin surface.
   b. Vein should appear ovoid in shape; transducer should be oblique to skin surface.
   c. Vein should fill screen from left to right; transducer should be perpendicular to skin surface.
   d. Vein should fill screen from left to right; transducer should be oblique to skin surface.

8. At what distance should marks be placed along the length of the vein when marking?
   a. 2 to 3 in
   b. 2 to 3 cm
   c. 5 to 6 cm
   d. 8 to 9 cm

9. When mapping and marking superficial veins, what is the transverse orientation useful to help identify?
   a. the relationship of superficial veins to deep veins
   b. branch points and vein diameter
   c. vein diameter only
   d. branch points and perforator location only

10. When measuring vein diameters for use as a conduit, how should the veins be measured?
    a. outer wall to outer wall
    b. outer wall to inner wall
    c. inner wall to outer wall
    d. inner wall to inner wall

11. In which part of the arm are the superficial veins easiest to identify?
    a. upper arm
    b. forearm
    c. near the wrist
    d. at the antecubital fossa

12. Why are the vessels easier to identify at the upper arm?
    a. The vessels are deeper and smaller in diameter.
    b. The vessels are larger and have the least amount of branches.
    c. The vessels are more superficial with multiple branches.
    d. The vessels follow the deep system.

13. Which landmark can be used to identify the cephalic vein in the upper arm?
    a. brachial artery
    b. radial artery
    c. biceps muscle
    d. clavicle

14. Which transducer frequency would be most appropriate for mapping of the cephalic vein?
    a. 7 MHz
    b. 3.5 MHz
    c. 10 MHz
    d. 15 MHz

15. During a vein mapping procedure, the technologist visualizes a portion of the great saphenous vein that is partially compressible with decreased phasicity upon Doppler interrogation. What does this most likely represent?
    a. acute, occlusive thrombosis
    b. partial thrombosis of the great saphenous vein section
    c. chronic thrombosis of a varicosity
    d. normal findings in the great saphenous vein

16. Which condition results in a vein that is unusable as a bypass conduit?
    a. wall thickening with evidence of recanalization
    b. vein wall calcifications
    c. isolated valve abnormalities
    d. all of the above ⟵

17. During a venous mapping procedure, the patient notes that she has had prior vein stripping; however, the technologist finds a large superficial vein on the anterior medial aspect of the thigh. What does this most likely represent?
    a. The main great saphenous vein, which has recanalized.
    b. The anterior accessory saphenous vein, which has become dominant.
    c. The posterior accessory saphenous vein, which has become dominant.
    d. A varicosity that should not be evaluated.

18. What minimum size is required for a vein to be used as a conduit?
    a. 1.0 to 2.0 mm
    b. 1.0 to 2.0 cm
    c. 2.5 to 3.0 mm
    d. 1.5 to 2.0 mm

19. During a venous mapping procedure, the technologist notes a thin, echogenic line protruding into the vessel lumen that does not appear to be mobile. The patient does not have a history of previous superficial thrombophlebitis. What does this finding likely represent?
    a. chronic thrombosis
    b. stenotic, frozen valve
    c. vein wall calcification
    d. varicosity

20. When using color and spectral Doppler to evaluate the superficial venous system, which settings should be used?
    a. high gain and high PRF/scale
    b. low gain and high PRF/scale
    c. low gain and low PRF/scale
    d. high gain and low PRF/scale

Fill-in-the-Blank

1. A common application for superficial venous mapping is to evaluate veins for use as lower extremity or coronary _artery bypass graft_

2. The _small saphenous_ vein is the standard name for the vein previously known as the lesser or short saphenous vein.

3. If the great saphenous vein has been removed, the _upper extremity_ systems may be a suitable alternative.

4. Venous mapping of the upper extremity veins is routine in the preoperative assessment for patients undergoing the creation of _AV fistula._

5. When using a superficial vein for in situ arterial bypass, _perforating_ veins must always be identified and ligated.

6. The cephalic vein courses up the _radial_ side of the forearm, whereas the basilic vein courses up the _ular_ side of the forearm.

7. The main great saphenous vein is typically bounded superficially by the _superficial facia_ and deeply by the _muscular facia_

8. There are several common configurations on the great saphenous vein. Most often, there is a _single_ trunk, which runs _medial_ in the thigh.

9. When a double saphenous system occurs, it is important to distinguish which system is _dominate_ so the surgeon can select appropriately.

10. The small saphenous vein is typically a single trunk that courses up the middle of the posterior aspect of the calf and terminates into the _popliteal_ vein.

11. When mapping directly onto the patient's skin, limited use of gel will allow easier marking on the skin and reduce the amount of _cooling_ the patient experiences because of gel evaporation.

12. The optimal patient position for mapping of the great saphenous vein is a _reverse trendelenburg_ position with the hip externally rotated and knee flexed.

13. When starting to map the great saphenous vein, it can be identified at the _saphenofemoral_ junction in a transverse orientation using light probe pressure.

14. If using a longitudinal approach to vein mapping, the technologist should be sure that the vein completely fills the screen from right to left and that the transducer is _perpendicular_ to the skin surface.

15. When mapping a vein, two types of branches should be identified: _cutaneous tributaries_ branches and deep _perforating_ veins.

16. Because of how vein diameters are measured, vein sizes are often _underestimated_ when compared to intraoperative measurements.

17. Appropriate system settings for venous mapping include adjusting the transmit power and focal zones for a well-defined _near_ field image and adjusting Doppler settings to detect _low flow veins_.

18. Keeping the patient warm during a vein mapping procedure helps to reduce peripheral _vasoconstriction_.

19. Diabetics and patients with end-stage renal disease can often have venous _calcification_ that may make a vein unsuitable for bypass material.

20. Veins presenting with an irregular intimal surface or wall thickening may indicate evidence of _recanalization_.

Short Answer

1. Describe the characteristics of a normal, healthy vein that may be used for mapping, including optimum diameter.

Smooth, thin walls, compliant & easily compressible. Have freely moving valve leaflets & diameter between 2.5 to 3 mm

2. What methods and techniques can be used to ensure a successful vein mapping procedure?

not too much gell. Mark in front of transducer & have the transducer perpendicular to the skin & mark every 2 to 3cm

IMAGE EVALUATION/PATHOLOGY

Review the images and answer the following questions.

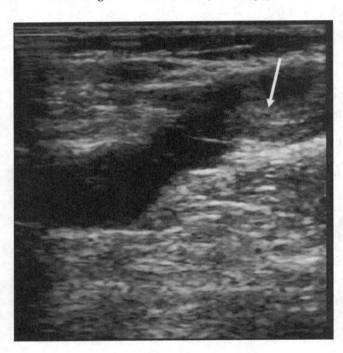

1. The image demonstrates the saphenofemoral junction. Describe the findings indicated by the white arrows.

valve leaflet with thrombus adjacent to it

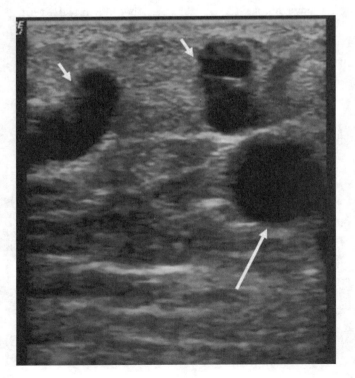

2. Describe the findings demonstrated on the image to the left. Would this vein be adequate for use as a conduit for arterial bypass?

Superficial varices with the main saphenous system beneath.
yes

CASE STUDY

Review the information and answer the following questions.

1. A 66-year-old male presents to the vascular lab for lower extremity vein mapping prior to right femoral–popliteal arterial bypass grafting. During the procedure, the right great saphenous vein demonstrates evidence of segmental chronic venous thrombosis. What options may the surgeon have in this case? What additional vessels would be appropriate to evaluate?

   The surgeon can find a part that doesn't have any thrombus in or use the small saphenous vein

2. You have completed a vein mapping procedure on a 75-year-old female and have the following findings: left great saphenous vein measures 2.8 to 3.3 mm in the thigh and 1.6 to 2.5 mm in the calf; right great saphenous vein measures 1.9 to 2.4 mm in the thigh and 1.3 to 1.9 mm in the calf; left small saphenous measures 0.9 to 1.2 mm; and right small saphenous measures 1.7 to 2.1 mm. Which vein segments would you recommend for use to your vascular surgeon for lower extremity bypass grafting? What techniques could be used to help ensure maximum dilation of the veins?

   left great sphenous vein
   maximize venous pressure
   put patient in reverse trendelenburg

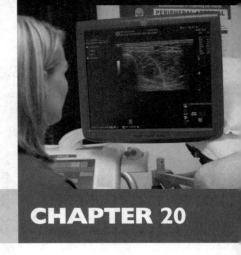

Venous Valvular Insufficiency Testing

REVIEW OF GLOSSARY TERMS

Matching

Match the key terms with their definitions.

KEY TERMS

1. _____ reticular veins

2. _____ varicose veins

3. _____ CEAP

4. _____ chronic venous insufficiency

5. _____ reflux

6. _____ lymphedema

7. _____ lipedema

8. _____ spider vein

9. _____ vein of Giacomini

10. _____ anterior accessory great saphenous vein

11. _____ great saphenous vein

12. _____ elastic compression

13. _____ leg edema

14. _____ nonsaphenous veins

15. _____ plethysmography

16. _____ posterior accessory saphenous vein

17. _____ small saphenous vein

18. _____ tributary vein

DEFINITION

a. Superficial vein at the posterior medial thigh

b. Swelling attributed to fat tissue

c. Clinical, etiologic, anatomic, and pathophysiologic classification of chronic venous insufficiency

d. Superficial vein at the anterior thigh

e. Small clusters of veins near the skin surface that may be red, blue, or purple, measuring between 0.5 and 1 mm; also known as telangiectasias

f. Veins with a diameter less than 3 mm

g. Superficial vein in the medial aspect of the lower extremity, thigh, and calf

h. Swelling attributed to lymph channels or lymph node disorders

i. Term attributed to the effects of stockings used to compress the leg with intent to compress the veins

j. Veins with diameter equal to or greater than 3 mm

k. Leg swelling

l. Long-lasting venous valvular or obstructive disorder

m. A vein that terminates or empties into another often larger vein

n. Reverse flow, usually in veins with incompetent valves

o. Superficial venous segments that are not part of the great and small saphenous systems

p. Communicating vein between the great and small saphenous veins

q. Graphic presentation of pulses such as changes in volume within an organ or other part of the body such as the lower extremity

r. Superficial vein in the posterior aspect of the calf

ANATOMY AND PHYSIOLOGY REVIEW

Image Labeling

Complete the labels in the images that follow.

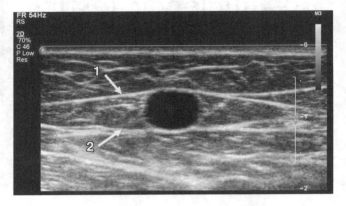

1. A transverse view through the mid-medial thigh.

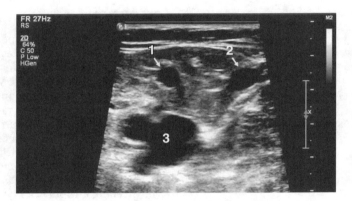

2. A transverse view at the proximal-medial thigh.

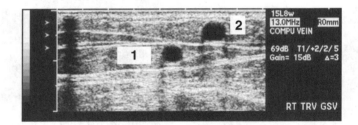

3. A transverse view through the mid-medial thigh.

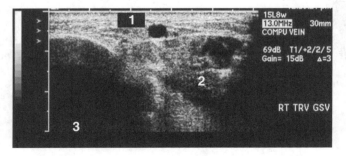

4. A transverse view through the medial proximal calf.

CHAPTER REVIEW

Multiple Choice

Complete each question by circling the best answer.

1. In which population are varicose veins typically more common?
   a. men
   b. women
   c. varicose veins occur as frequently in men as women
   d. men older than 65 years of age

2. What are other causes of leg edema that may mimic venous obstruction or valvular insufficiency?
   a. lymphatic obstruction
   b. cardiac disorders
   c. lipedema
   d. all the above

3. A patient presents to the vascular lab with visible spider veins. Based on this information, what would this patient's clinical CEAP classification likely be?
   a. C0
   b. C1
   c. C2
   d. C3

4. A patient presents to the vascular lab with chronic bilateral leg swelling. Upon duplex assessment of the venous system, the deep system was found to be unremarkable, although there was reflux demonstrated in the bilateral great saphenous veins. What is the most likely CEAP classification for this patient?
   a. C3EpAsPr
   b. C2EsApPo
   c. C3EcAsPro
   d. C6EpAsPro

5. Venous pressure in the legs in a supine individual is _____ mm Hg at its highest, whereas it increases to about _____ mm Hg with standing, depending on a person's height.
   a. 25, 200
   b. 10, 20
   c. 10, 100
   d. 50, 120

6. What is the reason for the increase in venous pressure with standing?
   a. cardiac pulsatility
   b. the effect of valves on venous flow
   c. systolic pressure gradients
   d. introduction of hydrostatic pressure

7. Within which of the following positions can a true saphenous vein be determined?
   a. deep muscular fascia
   b. subdural lipid layer
   c. saphenous fascia
   d. anterior vascular compartment

8. Which of the following is aligned with the deep system?
   a. anterior accessory saphenous vein
   b. great saphenous vein
   c. posterior accessory saphenous vein
   d. small saphenous vein

9. Into which of the following vessels does the small saphenous vein terminate?
   a. popliteal vein
   b. gastrocnemius vein
   c. distal femoral vein
   d. any of the above

10. Before assessing the venous system for insufficiency/reflux, which of the following should be performed?
    a. Evaluation of the deep venous system for obstruction or thrombosis
    b. Evaluation of the arterial system for atherosclerotic development
    c. Mapping of the superficial venous system
    d. Auscultation for bruits in the lower extremities

11. To best demonstrate valvular incompetence, which position should the patient be examined in?
    a. supine
    b. reverse Trendelenburg
    c. standing
    d. Trendelenburg

12. When performing an examination for CVVI, patency and flow characteristics should be documented at all the following locations EXCEPT:
    a. common femoral vein.
    b. femoral vein.
    c. popliteal vein.
    d. anterior tibial vein.

13. Which technique should be used to quantify reflux flow patterns?

    a. B-mode imaging with B flow

    b. color-flow Doppler

    c. spectral Doppler

    d. power Doppler

14. Pathologic flow or reflux occurs during _____ of an automatic cuff when the cuff is distal to the site of insonation.

    a. compression

    b. decompression

    c. application

    d. none of the above

15. Which of the following describes the proper use of an automatic cuff compression device?

    a. Rapid inflation from 70 to 80 mm Hg of pressure, held for a few seconds and released quickly.

    b. Paced inflation from 70 to 80 mm Hg of pressure, then released quickly.

    c. Rapid inflation from 120 to 150 mm Hg with immediate rapid deflation.

    d. Gradual inflation and deflation of the cuff with the patient's respiratory cycle.

16. What is the major advantage of using hand compression instead of automatic cuff inflators?

    a. reproducibility

    b. adaptability to unusual venous segments

    c. standardized technique and pressures

    d. less technical error

17. Which of the following is NOT a pitfall in measuring reflux?

    a. High persistence resulting in false-positive color-flow findings.

    b. High-velocity scale or PRF setting affecting color-flow sensitivity.

    c. Low-wall filter settings allowing visualization of low-velocity venous flow.

    d. Gain settings too high altering the sensitivity of spectral Doppler.

18. After thermal ablation of a vein, what do the sonographic findings include?

    a. smooth, thin-walled veins that are fully compressible with anechoic lumens

    b. dilated, incompressible veins with hypoechoic material filling the vein

    c. small-diameter vein that is partially compressible with an echogenic lumen

    d. potentially sonographically absent, fibrosed, or recanalized veins at different locations along the vein length

19. Valvular reflux times as measured on a spectral Doppler display are typically considered abnormal when greater than how many seconds?

    a. 1

    b. 2

    c. 3

    d. 4

20. What is the main purpose for venous photoplethysmography of the lower limb?

    a. Definitive diagnosis of venous reflux

    b. Determination of level of reflux

    c. Screening for detection of reflux

    d. Screening for venous thrombosis

21. What can the use of a tourniquet during venous PPG testing help determine?

    a. deep versus superficial venous reflux

    b. great saphenous versus accessory saphenous vein reflux

    c. venous reflux versus venous thrombosis

    d. perforating vein reflux

22. A patient presents to the vascular laboratory for evaluation of valvular incompetence. A venous PPG examination is performed. The results of the examination demonstrate a venous refill time (VRT) of 10.5 seconds without the use of a tourniquet and 22 seconds with the use of a tourniquet. What do these findings demonstrate?

    a. normal findings

    b. presence of deep venous reflux

    c. presence of superficial venous reflux

    d. presence of both deep and superficial venous reflux

23. What is air plethysmography useful for?

    a. Determining deep versus superficial venous thrombosis.

    b. Determining deep versus superficial venous reflux.

    c. Qualification of deep venous reflux.

    d. Quantification of chronic venous insufficiency.

24. Using APG, increased ambulatory pressures suggestive of the inability to empty the calf veins owing to poor or nonfunctional calf muscle pump are indicated with the which of the following findings?

    a. residual volume greater than 20% to 35%

    b. low venous volume

    c. venous filling rate less than 2 mL/s

    d. venous filling time greater than 25 seconds

25. Which of the following is an emerging technology that may help with guidance of venous access, phlebotomy, and injection sclerotherapy?
    a. venous photoplethysmography
    b. near-infrared imaging
    c. air plethysmography
    d. radio frequency imaging

Fill-in-the-Blank

1. Chronic venous insufficiency (CVI) is a term used to describe venous insufficiency due to venous _____ or _____ insufficiency.

2. Along with the great and small saphenous veins, the vascular technologist must also be familiar with the posterior and anterior _____ saphenous veins.

3. Saphenous veins are within a saphenous _____, readily identifying them on ultrasound. This structure gives the saphenous veins their distinctive _____ appearance.

4. The landmark to identify the anterior accessory saphenous vein is the _____, which is a vertical line perpendicular to the transducer surface that runs through the femoral artery and vein.

5. Veins that pierce the saphenous fascia and drain into another major vein are known as _____ veins.

6. The triangle formed by the gastrocnemius muscle, the tibial bone, and great saphenous vein used to identify the GSV below the knee is known as the "_____."

7. The tributary of the GSV near the saphenofemoral junction that is commonly used as a landmark for the venous ablation catheter is the _____ vein.

8. The confluence of the small saphenous vein and the deep venous system is _____, terminating into the popliteal vein, femoral vein, or other deep or perforating veins.

9. Normal venous valves allow for _____ flow direction, whereas incompetent valves permit _____ flow or reflux.

10. Prevalence of venous reflux tends to increase with the severity of _____ and with increasing _____.

11. Visual signs of abnormal venous pressures, such as spider veins or skin changes, are the primary basis for _____ classification.

12. Temporary leg swelling at the end of a working day, after prolonged standing, or as result of leg positioning, may represent _____.

13. Cardiac disease, arterial disease, sympathetic tone, or lipid disorders are all differential diagnoses for _____.

14. A skin change that results in a cluster of veins and skin changes, usually at the ankle, is _____.

15. A patient with open skin ulcers, CVVI as major cause of clinical manifestations, and affecting superficial and perforating veins with a pathologic combination of pathophysiology would have a CEAP classification of _____.

16. Duplex Doppler ultrasonography has two major diagnostic goals for CVVI: first is to rule out _____ and the second is the evaluation of _____ (reflux detection).

17. A concise duplex ultrasound evaluation designed for patients at risk or with a high probability of having CVVI is a _____ exam.

18. An invasive diagnostic method to detect venous thrombosis, congenital venous malformations, or valvular function is _____.

19. A CVVI treatment option which uses a foamed or liquid chemical agent injected directly into the vein is termed _____.

20. A popular treatment for CVVI which uses radio frequency or laser energy to close the affected veins is termed _____.

21. Patient positioning for evaluation for venous disease typically starts with the patient in _____ position for evaluation of deep veins, whereas a _____ position is recommended for evaluation of CVVI.

22. If on initial assessment of a patient with suspected CVVI acute DVT is detected, the continuation of the CVVI evaluation is _____.

23. When using proper compression techniques, abnormal veins proximal to the site of compression would demonstrate _____ flow during compression with _____ flow during decompression.

24. The most reproducible methods of compression include an automatic cuff and the "_____" maneuver.

25. Reflux time measurement should be performed with _____ Doppler with the vein in a sagittal image.

26. When performing a screening examination for CVVI, the scan can be interrupted after finding _____ level(s) of saphenous or nonsaphenous abnormality.

27. Evaluation of the femoropopliteal veins, deep calf veins, and entire superficial system (saphenous and nonsaphenous veins) would be appropriate in the _____ diagnosis of CVVI.

28. During thermal ablation treatment of CVVI, selection of incision site, insertion of needles, introducers, guide wires, and catheters and placement of tumescent anesthesia are all performed under _____.

29. During postablation follow-up, the most important ultrasound documentation should be of the _____ veins to assure patency.

30. To optimize detection of reflux, system settings such as gain, scale/PRF, and persistence, should be adjusted to detect _____.

31. In the diagnosis of CVVI, the measurement of reflux _____ is commonly preferred to measurement of peak reverse velocity or reflux volume flow rate.

32. In venous photoplethysmography, a PPG transducer is placed on the _____ aspect of the calf and venous _____ time is measured after the patient performs 5 to 10 foot flexion maneuvers.

33. Air plethysmography (APG) is a recommended technique for _____ of chronic venous insufficiency.

34. In APG studies, patient performance of a series of maneuvers is _____ in obtaining reliable results.

35. A patient with a filling time (FT) of >25 seconds, filling rate (FR) <2 mL/s, and a residual volume (RV) <20% would be considered _____ with respect to CVVI.

Short Answer

1. What are the typical symptoms associated with valvular insufficiency?

2. Other than CEAP classification, what are the other clinical evaluation tools designed to help quantify and describe the effects of venous valvular insufficiency on a patient's daily life?

3. What is a recommended order of evaluation of lower extremity venous segments to help optimize the standing examination?

4. How is color Doppler used in the diagnosis of CVVI?

5. What is the role of photoplethysmography and air plethysmography in the diagnosis of CVVI?

IMAGE EVALUATION/PATHOLOGY

Review the images and answer the following questions.

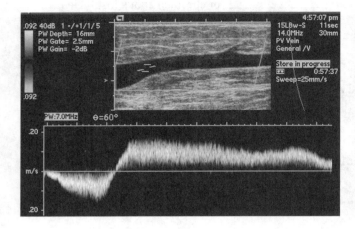

1. This image was taken in the great saphenous vein just distal to the saphenofemoral junction. The patient was asked to perform a Valsalva maneuver, and this image was the result. Explain the findings and if they are significant.

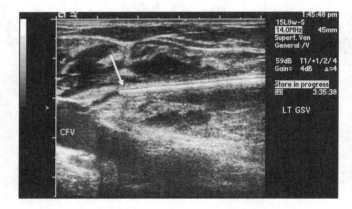

2. This image is of the left great saphenous vein just distal to the saphenofemoral junction. Describe the structure the white arrow is pointing to. What is its purpose?

CASE STUDY

Review the information and answer the following questions.

1. A 44-year-old female presents to the vascular lab with the CEAP classification, C2EpAsPr. She has been referred for verification of this classification by duplex testing. Explain the CEAP classification for this patient. What duplex protocol would be most appropriate for this patient, and what would you expect the findings to be?

2. A 52-year-old female presents to the vascular lab for varicose vein evaluation. Findings during the evaluation were as follows:
   - Right GSV: visually enlarged and tortuous with retrograde flow lasting 750 ms, retrograde flow also visualized with color throughout entire length.
   - Left GSV: visually appears to have normal diameter; minimal retrograde flow (<350 ms).

- Right femoropopliteal segments: thickened vessel walls with mostly anechoic lumens that are not fully compressible with transducer compression and retrograde flow noted at 1.2 seconds.
- Left femoropopliteal segments: anechoic lumens that are compressible with transducer compression with minimal retrograde flow (<0.5 seconds).

Which vessel(s) demonstrate reflux? Of the vessels that demonstrate reflux, what is the likely underlying pathophysiology?

3. A 67-year-old male presents to the vascular lab for venous APG testing. A standard APG test is performed with the following results:

Venous volume = 200 mL

Venous filling time = 10 seconds

Venous filling rate = 2.5 mL/s

Residual volume percentage = 37%

What do these results suggest? What further testing, if any, should be suggested in this patient?

Sonography in the Venous Treatment Room

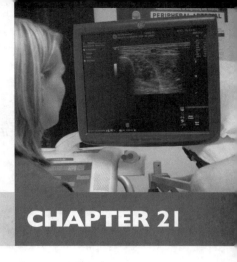

REVIEW OF GLOSSARY TERMS

Matching

Match the key terms with their definitions.

KEY TERMS

1. _____ endovenous ablation

2. _____ chronic venous insufficiency

3. _____ phlebologist

4. _____ reflux

5. _____ sclerosant

6. _____ sclerotherapy

7. _____ perivenous (tumescent) anesthesia

DEFINITION

a. A medical procedure involving an injection of a sclerosant into the vein. May be performed visually or under ultrasound guidance

b. Physician who specializes in the diagnosis and treatment of vein disorders

c. Anesthesia that is placed around the vein to be treated with thermal ablation under ultrasound guidance

d. Destruction of the vein by various means (e.g., heat, chemical)

e. A chemical irritant used in the treatment of varicose veins resulting in inflammation and subsequent fibrosis, thus obliterating the lumen of the vein

f. A long-lasting venous valvular or obstructive disorder of the veins

g. Pathologic condition in a vein defined as retrograde flow upon release of distal compression in a standing patient

CHAPTER REVIEW

Multiple Choice

Complete each question by circling the best answer.

1. Which of the following are reasons why traditional surgical stripping and ligation are rarely performed?
   a. invasive and painful procedure
   b. requires general anesthesia
   c. prolonged recovery requiring weeks to months
   d. all the above

2. What is the surgical procedure in which a small incision is created next to a varicosity and a special instrument is used to hook and extract the vein?
   a. chemical ablation
   b. endovenous thermal ablation
   c. ambulatory phlebectomy
   d. stripping and ligation

3. Which of the following is a credential that can be earned to demonstrate a thorough knowledge of venous anatomy and hemodynamics?
   a. ARNP
   b. RPhS
   c. RCS
   d. RVT

4. What is the primary role of the sonographer in the intervention room during venous treatment?
   a. Provide ultrasound guidance.
   b. Make clinical decisions regarding treatment.
   c. Perform chemical ablation procedures.
   d. Provide patient care during the procedure.

5. Which of the following would be a critical step in preparing the patient for a venous treatment procedure?
   a. Documenting the patient's clinical condition
   b. Verifying the correct leg and vein to be treated
   c. Scheduling a postoperative appointment
   d. Explaining the venous disease process

6. When the small saphenous vein is being treated, what is the most common patient position used to ensure access to this vein?
   a. reverse Trendelenburg
   b. Trendelenburg
   c. supine
   d. prone

7. Because of the location of most of the veins that will be evaluated in the intervention room, what are the typical transducer frequencies that will be used?
   a. low frequency
   b. intermediate frequency
   c. high frequency
   d. ultra-low frequency

8. While providing ultrasound guidance, what is indicated by a vein that has a notably thickened wall and a reduced lumen diameter?
   a. acute thrombosis
   b. vasospasm
   c. chronic thrombosis
   d. arterialization

9. What is the advantage of viewing the access needle in a longitudinal plane rather than transverse?
   a. View of needle over the medial or lateral portion of the vein
   b. Inability to apply pressure on the vein
   c. Needle can be more easily advanced directly under the transducer
   d. Ability to determine whether the needle has punctured the posterior vein wall

10. What is the term for blood that is returned through the needle when accessing a vein?
    a. flash
    b. core of tissue
    c. rush
    d. streak

11. Where should the guidewire be located?
    a. between the vein and the superficial fascia
    b. intraluminally in the vein to be treated
    c. between the vein and the deep fascia
    d. extravascular

12. What landmark should be used to ensure the tip of the treatment device is positioned appropriately in the great saphenous vein?
    a. preterminal valve of the GSV
    b. external pudendal vein
    c. superficial epigastric vein
    d. anterior accessory saphenous vein

13. Which structure is near the saphenopopliteal junction and can be injured by the treatment device?
    a. gastrocnemius vein
    b. superior epigastric vein
    c. peroneal nerve
    d. sciatic verve

14. Once the treatment device is in place, what position should the patient be placed in before treatment begins, ensuring the veins empty and contract around the device?
    a. Trendelenburg
    b. reverse Trendelenburg
    c. prone
    d. left lateral decubitus

15. Which imaging plane is typically preferred for guidance of placement of tumescent anesthesia?
    a. transverse
    b. longitudinal
    c. posterior oblique
    d. coronal

16. After placing the tumescent anesthesia, what is the minimum separation between the treated vein and the skin line?
    a. 1 to 2 cm
    b. 2 to 4 cm
    c. 4 to 6 cm
    d. 8 to 10 cm

17. What would a hyperechoic echo actively forming as the thermal ablation device is being withdrawn represent?
    a. active acute thrombosis
    b. injection of tumescent anesthesia
    c. destruction of the endothelial lining
    d. laser energy from the thermal catheter

18. When should initial follow-up occur after a patient has had thermal ablation?
    a. within 1 to 2 hours
    b. 14 to 20 days postprocedure
    c. 1 month postprocedure
    d. 2 to 7 days postprocedure

19. When administering a chemical sclerosing agent, what is the optimum patient position to visualize the veins and flow abnormalities?
    a. reverse Trendelenburg
    b. Trendelenburg
    c. standing
    d. supine

20. Which of the following is typically applied to the patient's leg postablation procedure?
    a. small bandages over incision sites and graduated compression stockings
    b. small bandages over incision sites and nothing else
    c. soft, supportive cast
    d. absorbent pads and bandages over incision sites

Fill-in-the-Blank

1. The invasive, surgical, traditional treatment of chronic venous insufficiency is known as vein _____.

2. Current minimally invasive techniques for treatment of chronic venous insufficiency are largely performed under ultrasound _____ in order to place needles, devices, and drugs.

3. Treatment of bulbous tributaries, smaller varicosities, reticular veins, and telangiectasias typically involves _____ ablation.

4. A complication that may result during thermal ablation or administration of perivenous anesthesia because of a needle piercing both an artery and a vein is _____.

5. If a patient is scheduled for micro-phlebectomy, it is recommended that they remain standing for _____ minutes to ensure maximum distention of superficial veins.

6. While in the intervention room, ultrasound evaluation is primarily a(n) _____ procedure.

7. In preparation for an ablation procedure, many centers will _____ the vein to be treated so that it can be easily identified and followed.

8. A patient who is cold, dehydrated, or apprehensive about the interventional procedure may have veins that are in _____.

9. To maintain a sterile field during an ultrasound-guided procedure in the intervention room, the ultrasound transducer is placed in a(n) _____.

10. When gaining access to the vein for treatment, it is preferable to access below any large _____ to isolate their connection with truncal veins.

11. To help induce vasodilatation, heat or _____ can be applied.

12. After the guidewire is placed, a(n) _____ sheath is placed through which the ablation device will be introduced.

13. Encountering a valve or small tortuosity can cause _____ when advancing the catheter or treatment fiber.

14. When treating the small saphenous vein, the treatment device should not be advanced out of the _____.

15. On the ultrasound image, the tumescent anesthesia appears as a(n) _____ "cocoon" of fluid encircling the vein.

16. If the thermal ablation catheter is too close to the skin line, superficial _____ can occur and be permanent.

17. Pressure should be applied over a thermal ablation device to ensure that the vessel walls are _____ and in contact with the device.

18. Particularly large venous segments or connections with large tributaries warrant additional _____ and increased transducer pressure to ensure adequate closure.

19. To ensure a sclerosing agent completely fills the varicosities, the _____ from the cluster of treated vessels should be identified.

20. Adequate dispersion of a sclerosant can be accomplished by applying pressure or "_____" the tissues to move the sclerosant in the desired direction.

Short Answer

1. What are some methods that can be used in the intervention room to prevent vasospasm?

2. What are some methods that can be used to maintain a sterile field in the intervention room?

3. What complications may arise if the treatment device is not properly positioned at the terminal point?

4. What is the purpose of tumescent anesthesia?

IMAGE EVALUATION/PATHOLOGY

Review the images and answer the following questions.

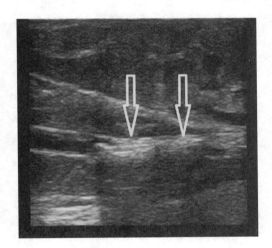

1. What is indicated by the arrows in this image?

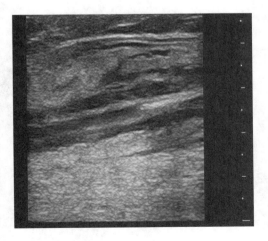

2. What is demonstrated by the hypoechoic area on either side of the vein?

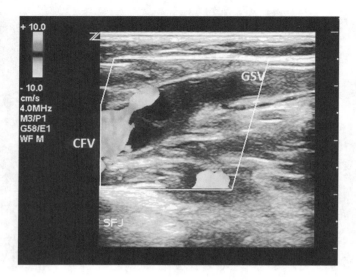

3. What is demonstrated in this image taken 3 days after great saphenous vein thermal ablation?

CASE STUDY

Review the information and answer the following questions.

1. A patient returns to the vascular lab 5 days after thermal ablation of the great saphenous vein. Upon follow-up examination, hypoechoic material is noted in the dilated GSV as well as the common femoral vein. The patient's peritreatment ultrasound exam is reviewed, and it is determined that the catheter tip was placed less than 1 cm from the superficial epigastric vein. What is likely happening in this patient and what is the cause?

2. A patient presents to the venous treatment center for thermal ablation. During ultrasound guidance of the placement of the perivenous anesthesia, it is noted that the anesthesia is not completely surrounding the vein and that the vein is less than 1 cm from the skin surface. If not corrected, what complications could occur in this patient?

The Role of Ultrasound in Central Vascular Access Device Placement

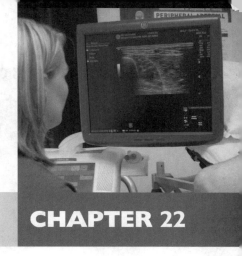

REVIEW OF GLOSSARY TERMS

Matching

Match the key terms with their definitions.

KEY TERMS

1. _____ air embolism

2. _____ fistula

3. _____ guidewire

4. _____ infiltration

5. _____ microintroducer

6. _____ PICC

7. _____ pneumothorax

8. _____ sheath

9. _____ stenosis

10. _____ peel-away sheath

11. _____ collateral vein

12. _____ gain

13. _____ guidewire

14. _____ intima

DEFINITION

a. A sheath that is perforated along the long axis, allowing device to be split for removal from a catheter

b. Preexisting veins which enlarge to take flow from neighboring but occluded vessels

c. A nitinol or stainless-steel wire used to support sheath or catheter exchanges and to predict vessel patency

d. Small needles and wires used to make the initial access into a target

e. Innermost layer of a vein or an artery; composed of one layer of endothelial cells in contact with blood flow

f. Narrowing of a vein or an artery due to disease or trauma

g. Collection of air in the pleural space (between the lung and the chest wall)

h. The brightness of an ultrasound image, which can be manipulated on most devices

i. An abnormal connection or passageway between two organs or vessels, may be created due to trauma or intentionally for therapeutic purposes

j. A thin-walled, hollow plastic tube through which wires and catheters can be advanced

k. A hydrophilic guidewire

l. Inadvertent release of air or gas into the venous system

m. A peripherally inserted central catheter; a type of vascular access device that is typically inserted into a vein of the upper extremity and threaded to achieve a tip location in the distal third of the superior vena cava

n. Leaking of IV fluid from a catheter into the tissue surrounding the vein

ANATOMY AND PHYSIOLOGY REVIEW

Image Labeling

Complete the labels in the images that follow.

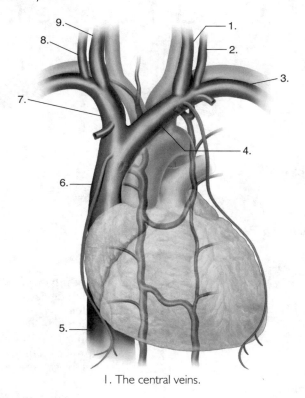

1. The central veins.

CHAPTER REVIEW

Multiple Choice

Complete each question by circling the best answer.

1. Central venous access may be used in patients requiring which of the following?
   a. intravenous antibiotic therapy
   b. chemotherapy
   c. total parenteral nutrition
   d. all the above

2. Which of the following is NOT one of the most commonly used peripheral access points for VAD placement?
   a. basilic vein
   b. cephalic vein
   c. popliteal vein
   d. internal jugular vein

3. Why is the atriocaval junction a desirable location for placement of the VAD catheter tip?
   a. Flow rates are around 2,000 mL/min.
   b. Blood flows directly into the left atrium from this location.
   c. Flow rates are typically lower for better dispersion.
   d. The atriocaval junction is NOT a desirable location.

4. What is a type of VAD that is placed percutaneously into a central or peripheral vein with its end secured at the puncture site?
   a. tunneled central VAD
   b. nontunneled central VAD
   c. implanted port
   d. port-a-cath

5. Which of the following is a type of VAD in which the catheter exits the skin away from the puncture site?
   a. tunneled central VAD
   b. nontunneled central VAD
   c. implanted port
   d. port-a-cath

6. Which of the following is NOT a benefit of a tunneled central VAD?
   a. reduction of device-related infection
   b. more stable device
   c. hidden exit site for cosmetic reasons
   d. less comfortable for the patient

7. Implanted ports are typically used in patients who require therapy at what rate?
   a. daily
   b. weekly
   c. every few hours
   d. continuously

8. Which of the following veins is typically the first choice for placement of peripherally inserted central catheters (PICCs)?
   a. cephalic vein
   b. brachial vein
   c. basilic vein
   d. axillary vein

9. For which of the following patients would it be more common to use the saphenous vein for central vascular access placement?
   a. a 75-year-old woman
   b. a 2-day-old infant
   c. a 35-year-old male
   d. a 62-year-old male

10. Which of the following describes the preferred use of peripheral cannulas?
    a. long-term (more than 1 year), continuous therapy
    b. long-term, intermittent therapy
    c. therapy lasting several months
    d. short-term therapy (less than 1 week)

11. Which jugular vein is preferred for central VAD placement?
    a. right internal jugular vein
    b. left internal jugular vein
    c. right external jugular vein
    d. left external jugular vein

12. Where is the internal jugular vein typically located in relation to the common carotid artery?
    a. directly lateral
    b. directly anterior
    c. anterolateral
    d. anteromedial

13. Because of their location around the clavicle, which of the following vessels is more difficult to visualize with ultrasound?
    a. axillary vein
    b. subclavian vein
    c. internal jugular vein
    d. basilic vein

14. Which of the following is a reason to avoid use of the common femoral vein in VAD placement?
    a. difficult to visualize on ultrasound
    b. preservation for use for lower extremity bypass grafting
    c. low-flow rates
    d. higher rate of mechanical and infectious complications

15. Which of the following is NOT included in the initial assessment for potential access sites for VAD placement?
    a. patency of the vessel
    b. location of vessel in relation to other structures
    c. blood flow velocity
    d. ability to access the target vessel

16. How is confirmation of tip placement of a vascular access device typically made?
    a. ultrasound
    b. chest x-ray
    c. CT scan
    d. contrast MRA

17. A patient presents to the vascular lab after VAD placement to evaluate the basilic vein in which the device is placed. Upon ultrasound evaluation, the basilic vein is noted to have an irregular intimal surface with low-level echoes within the vein lumen. What do these findings suggest?
    a. nontarget puncture and hematoma
    b. air embolism in the basilic vein
    c. vein damage with thrombosis
    d. arteriovenous fistula

18. Which of the following is one of the most serious and potentially life-threatening complications of central venous catheterization?
    a. pneumothorax
    b. arteriovenous fistula
    c. thrombosis
    d. vein wall damage

19. Which medication would be associated with an increased risk of bleeding during vascular access device placement?
    a. Clopidrogel
    b. Warfarin
    c. Heparin
    d. All the above

20. Which complication of VAD placement is often transient and results in few, if any, symptoms?
    a. vein wall damage
    b. cardiac arrhythmias
    c. arteriovenous fistula
    d. pneumothorax

Fill-in-the-Blank

1. Common target veins for central vascular access devices include _____ veins, such as the basilic and cephalic veins.

2. More centrally located target veins include the _____ and internal _____ veins.

3. The catheter tip of a vascular access device typically resides in the distal third of the _____ at the atriocaval junction.

4. A vascular access device designed to remain in place long term would be a _____ device.

5. Vascular access devices with a catheter segment attached to a plastic or titanium reservoir are _____.

6. Because of the location of the brachial veins next to the brachial artery, there is a higher risk of _____ if the brachial veins are used for peripheral VAD placement.

7. When accessing the central veins for central VAD placement, the _____ internal jugular vein is preferred because of a straighter course to the heart.

8. Ultrasound allows for _____ assessment of the internal jugular vein prior to VAD placement as well as dynamic guidance during vein puncture.

9. Using ultrasound guidance during vein puncture can reduce failure of catheter placement as well as complication rates related to _____.

10. When accessing the internal jugular vein, it is important to identify the _____ prior to attempting cannulation to avoid serious injury.

11. Neither the subclavian nor other upper extremity veins should be used for cannulation in patients with _____ to preserve these vessels for hemodialysis in the future.

12. The _____ veins are typically only used for venous access in emergent situations and in patients in whom other potential access veins are occluded.

13. Patency of a vessel for potential access is first tested by _____, similar to that used in the assessment of a patient for deep venous thrombosis.

14. On ultrasound, the VAD appears in the lumen of the vein and produces a(n) _____ structure on the image.

15. The presence of _____ veins upon physical examination should alert the clinician to potential difficulties in successful placement of VADs.

16. Thrombosis and arteriovenous fistula formation are examples of complications due to _____.

17. To minimize the impact of _____ puncture, a small access needle should be used.

18. Difficult or traumatic VAD insertion, hematologic disorders, and concurrent treatment with certain medications all increase the risk of _____ during VAD placement.

19. Using valved sheaths, performing exchange maneuvers efficiently, and assuring that catheter lumens are flushed, secured, and locked will decrease the risk of _____.

20. When advancing guidewires into the heart during VAD placement, transient, asymptomatic _____ often occur.

Short Answer

1. What are the factors that influence the matching of a patient to an appropriate vascular access device?

2. What is the difference between nontunneled and tunneled central vascular access devices?

3. Describe the scanning technique and key uses of ultrasound guidance during vascular access device placement.

IMAGE EVALUATION/PATHOLOGY

Review the images and answer the following questions.

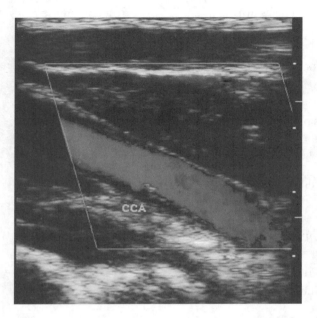

1. This image was taken from the proximal neck. What are these findings consistent with?

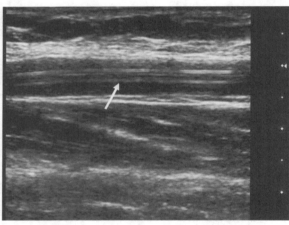

2. This image was taken in the mid-medial upper arm. What is shown in this image? Does this appear normal or abnormal?

CASE STUDY

Review the information and answer the following questions.

1. A 63-year-old female presents for evaluation of a central vascular access device that was placed through the internal jugular vein. A pulsatile mass was noted in the patient's neck. With this limited clinical information, what would the most likely cause of the pulsatile mass be, and what would be expected on the ultrasound examination?

2. A 57-year-old male presents for ultrasound evaluation after subclavian vein VAD placement. On the ultrasound examination, a hypoechoic area is noted adjacent to the subclavian vein. What are these findings consistent with, and what complications may arise?

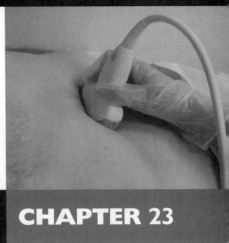

PART SIX

ABDOMINAL

Aorta and Iliac Arteries

CHAPTER 23

REVIEW OF GLOSSARY TERMS

Matching

Match the key terms with their definitions.

KEY TERMS

1. _____ aneurysm

2. _____ fusiform

3. _____ saccular

4. _____ endoleak

5. _____ endovascular aneurysm repair

6. _____ stent

DEFINITION

a. Asymmetric outpouching dilations of a vessel, often caused by trauma or penetrating aortic ulcers

b. Persistent blood flow demonstrated outside a stent graft endovascular repair but within aneurysm sac

c. A focal dilation of an artery involving all three layers of the vessel wall that exceeds the normal diameter by more than 50%

d. Placement of a stent graft within an aortic aneurysm sac via a catheter as a means of repair

e. Circumferential dilation of a vessel involving all three vessel walls

f. A tube-like structure placed inside a blood vessel to provide patency and support

ANATOMY AND PHYSIOLOGY REVIEW

Image Labeling

Complete the labels in the images that follow.

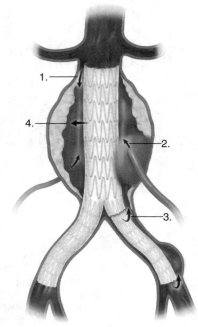

1. The types of endoleaks.

CHAPTER REVIEW

Multiple Choice

Complete each question by circling the best answer.

1. At about what rate are popliteal aneurysms associated with abdominal aortic aneurysms?

   a. 10%

   b. 20%

   c. 30%

   d. 50%

2. In which of the following patients would an abdominal aortic aneurysm most likely be found?

   a. a 69-year-old male

   b. a 75-year-old female

   c. a 37-year-old male

   d. a 28-year-old female

3. What causes the indication to evaluate the aortoiliac segments known as blue toe syndrome?

   a. vasospasm

   b. small vessel occlusive disease

   c. cold sensitivity

   d. embolic events

4. Which of the following patient preparation steps should be taken to reduce overlying bowel gas before an aortoiliac duplex evaluation?

   a. Take medication for gas reduction.

   b. Fast overnight.

   c. No specific preparation is necessary.

   d. Chew gum.

5. What position can the sonographer assume to help relieve strain on the arm and/or elbow when applying pressure to view the aorta and iliac arteries?

   a. Position shoulder over the transducer to allow body weight to help push.

   b. Abduct arm to reach across the patient.

   c. Bend at waist and extend arm to better visualize iliac vessels.

   d. Position flexed wrist over transducer and push from the shoulder.

6. To visualize the deep vessels of the abdomen, what transducer frequency is most commonly used?
   a. 7 to 10 MHz
   b. 2 to 5 MHz
   c. 5 to 8 MHz
   d. 1 to 2 MHz

7. What is the most common location for abdominal aortic aneurysms?
   a. suprarenal
   b. at the level of the superior mesenteric artery
   c. infrarenal
   d. proximal aorta just as it passes through the diaphragm

8. Which of the following is NOT associated with normal findings in the abdominal aorta?
   a. smooth margins
   b. tapering distally
   c. tortuosity near the bifurcation
   d. no focal dilatation

9. At what diameter is the abdominal aorta considered aneurysmal?
   a. 1 cm
   b. 2 cm
   c. 3 cm
   d. 3 mm

10. What shape are most aortic aneurysms?
    a. fusiform
    b. saccular
    c. mycotic
    d. dissecting

11. As an abdominal aortic aneurysm enlarges, what does it also tend to do?
    a. elongate
    b. foreshorten
    c. straighten
    d. constrict

12. To get the most accurate diameter measurement of the abdominal aorta, how should the technologist align the transducer to the vessel?
    a. parallelly
    b. obliquely
    c. perpendicularly
    d. sagittally

13. When viewing the abdominal aorta in transverse, which dimension provides the most accurate diameter measurement?
    a. anterior to posterior
    b. right to left lateral
    c. superior to inferior
    d. All are equally accurate.

14. During an aortoiliac duplex examination, the distal aorta measures 2.5 cm in diameter. What are these findings consistent with?
    a. normal aortic dimension
    b. aortic ectasia
    c. aortic aneurysm
    d. aortic dissection

15. When an abdominal aortic aneurysm is found, which of the following additional parameters should be included?
    a. length of aneurysm
    b. proximity of aneurysm to renal arteries
    c. presence and extent of any intraluminal thrombus
    d. all the above

16. What landmark is used to determine the end of the common iliac artery and beginning of the external iliac artery?
    a. inguinal ligament
    b. origin of internal iliac artery
    c. umbilicus
    d. iliac crest

17. What is an important reason to follow up with patients after aortoiliac intervention with duplex ultrasound?
    a. Follow-up and treatment of restenosis may improve patency rates.
    b. Occlusion is easier to manage than stenosis.
    c. Angioplasty and stenting do not have significant restenosis rates.
    d. Duplex ultrasound is not used for follow-up.

18. When evaluating a stent within the aortoiliac system, which of the following is FALSE?
    a. Stent alignment should be visualized.
    b. Full deployment of stent should be documented.
    c. Relationship of stent to vessel wall is needed.
    d. Evaluation of the vessel distal to the stent is not needed.

19. A 65-year-old male presents to the vascular lab for evaluation of the abdomen after involvement in a car accident. During the duplex examination, an asymmetric outpouching is identified in the mid to distal aorta. What do these findings represent?

    a. fusiform aneurysm

    b. saccular aneurysm

    c. aortic dissection

    d. aortic stenosis

20. Upon duplex evaluation of a known abdominal aortic aneurysm, homogeneous echoes with smooth borders are visualized with the aneurysm sac. What do these findings suggest?

    a. calcifications

    b. atherosclerotic plaque

    c. thrombus formation

    d. vessel dissection

21. A 72-year-old male presents to the vascular lab for follow-up after common iliac stenting. Upon examination, the stent in the mid common iliac artery is elliptical in shape. What does this appearance likely indicate?

    a. partial stent compression

    b. normally deployed stent

    c. a kink within the stent

    d. vessel dissection in the area of the stent

22. During Doppler evaluation of the abdominal aorta, two flow channels are noted. What do these findings suggest?

    a. fusiform aneurysm

    b. saccular aneurysm

    c. aortic dissection

    d. aortic stenosis

23. A 76-year-old female patient presents to the vascular lab with left hip and buttock claudication. During the duplex evaluation, velocities in the distal common iliac artery are 72 cm/s, whereas velocities in the proximal external iliac artery are 302 cm/s. Which of the following has occurred?

    a. >50% stenosis in the proximal external iliac artery

    b. <50% stenosis in the proximal external iliac artery

    c. >50% in the distal common iliac artery

    d. external iliac artery dissection

24. Which of the following is NOT a benefit of endovascular stent graft repair of AAA?

    a. lower perioperative mortality

    b. decreased survival rates over open surgical repair

    c. shorter recovery time

    d. lack of abdominal incision

25. What is the goal of EVAR?

    a. Reduce the size of the aortic lumen.

    b. Occlude the aorta to avoid aortic rupture.

    c. Exclude the aneurysm sac from the general circulation.

    d. Increase the size of the aorta to treat stenosis.

26. Which of the following can color Doppler ultrasound monitoring of EVAR demonstrate?

    a. residual sac size

    b. graft limb dysfunction and kinking

    c. hemodynamics within the graft site

    d. all the above

27. Which of the following is the most frequently deployed stent graft device?

    a. bifurcated

    b. straight tube

    c. uni-iliac graft

    d. fenestrated grafts

28. During the evaluation of an aortic stent graft, the vascular technologist notes a hyperechoic signal along the anterior and posterior walls of the aortic lumen just below the level of the renal arteries. What does this finding suggest?

    a. kinking of the stent graft

    b. normal findings of the proximal attachment site

    c. endoleak at the proximal graft site

    d. graft bifurcation at the distal attachment site

29. Which of the following is NOT an indication of aneurysm sac instability after EVAR?

    a. increase in sac size

    b. pulsatility of the sac

    c. decrease in size of aneurysm sac

    d. areas of echolucency within the sac

30. An 80-year-old male presents for follow-up after endovascular treatment of his AAA. During the evaluation, the stent graft is identified and appears to be in a correct position by B-mode; however, the aortic diameter is 5.5 cm compared to 4.9 cm on previous examination. Doppler evaluation is then performed, and flow is identified along the posterior aorta outside the stent graft material. What is the likely cause of these findings?

    a. kinking of the stent graft material

    b. stent graft endoleak

    c. migration of the stent graft causing stenosis

    d. normal findings after stent graft placement

Fill-in-the-Blank

1. The incidence of AAA in the United States is _____, and it is the _____ leading cause of death.

2. In preparation for aortoiliac duplex, the patient should _____ to minimize the effects of bowel gas.

3. A helpful patient position that can be used when an anteroposterior approach is obscured by abdominal contents, bowel gas, or scar tissue is _____.

4. Ultrasound evaluation of the aorta and iliac vessels should begin at the level of the _____ and extend to the _____ bifurcation.

5. The normal aorta tapers distally and terminates at the level of the _____.

6. When performing diameter measurements of the aorta, care must be taken to ensure that the transducer is _____ to the aorta itself, especially in the event of aortic neck angulation.

7. In addition to documenting aortic diameter and length, it is important to note the proximity to the _____ arteries because this will play a role in treatment decisions.

8. All spectral Doppler waveforms are collected maintaining an angle of _____ degrees or less and _____ to the vessel wall.

9. During preintervention evaluation of the aortoiliac segments, differentiation of disease proximal or distal to the _____ is important in the management of patients with lower extremity ischemia.

10. Following intervention, duplex follow-up becomes important because percutaneous angioplasty and stent procedures are associated with significant _____ rates.

11. When assessing a patient after PTA and/or stenting, it is important to image several centimeters _____ the treated area as well as through the treated area.

12. Because the iliac vessels are typically deep and tortuous, _____ Doppler is often useful to visualize these vessels to help obtain proper angle alignment.

13. Aortic _____ is present when the aorta demonstrates irregular margins and a nontapering profile.

14. Iliac arteries are considered aneurysmal when the diameter increases more than _____% compared to an adjacent segment or generally when the diameter exceeds _____ cm.

15. A complication of iliac artery aneurysms that results in dilation of the collecting system of the kidney is _____.

16. A(n) _____ may appear as a small, isolated wall defect where a short piece of the vessel wall protrudes into the vessel lumen.

17. _____ occurs when a tear forms between layers of the vessel wall, usually the intima–media interface, forming a false lumen.

18. A(n) _____ within a stent may appear as a sharp angulation of the stent walls in an otherwise straight vessel segment.

19. When evaluating the hemodynamics in the aorta, the proximal aorta demonstrates _____-resistance characteristics, whereas the distal aorta demonstrates _____-resistance characteristics.

20. When evaluating arterial hemodynamics, severe proximal disease results in turbulence and/or _____ in the distal signals.

21. Chronic _____ in the iliac arterial system can be difficult to visualize because the artery can become contracted and echogenic.

22. _____ repair of AAA is a less invasive procedure with lower perioperative mortality rates and shorter recovery time when compared to the traditional method.

23. Close surveillance is mandatory after EVAR because _____ is still possible if an endoleak is present.

24. An important benefit of color duplex ultrasound evaluation of an aortic stent graft is the ability to provide _____ information that is not available with other imaging modalities.

25. When a fenestrated graft is used for EVAR, it is important to document the patency of the _____ arteries after stent deployment.

26. Hypoechogenicity or heterogeneity with a spongy texture of the residual aneurysm sac may be associated with _____.

27. A key to identifying endoleak is a spectral Doppler flow pattern that is _____ from the aortic endograft.

28. An unstable AAA sac where the aneurysm continues to expand because of persistent or recurrent pressurization in the absence of endoleak is termed _____.

29. _____ Doppler can facilitate the detection of low-flow amplitude endoleaks that may course off-axis to the main sound beam.

30. The use of _____ imaging can facilitate the identification of the attachment sites and characterize thrombus within the residual sac by improving overall quality and contrast resolution of the image.

Short Answer

1. What are the common indications for performance of an aortoiliac duplex examination?

2. During preintervention duplex assessment of the aortoiliac segments, what can be determined on the duplex ultrasound images?

3. What are the common technical considerations and pitfalls associated with evaluation of the aorta and iliac vessels?

4. What is the role of color duplex ultrasound imaging in EVAR surveillance?

IMAGE EVALUATION/PATHOLOGY

Review the images and answer the following questions.

1. The images were taken from the right external iliac artery. What are your findings?

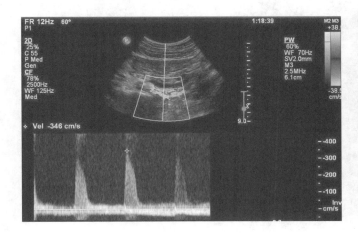 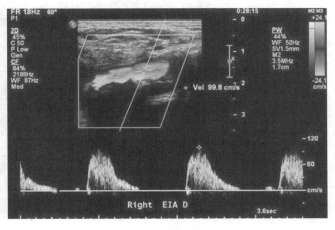

2. These images were taken on follow-up of EVAR. Describe the findings.

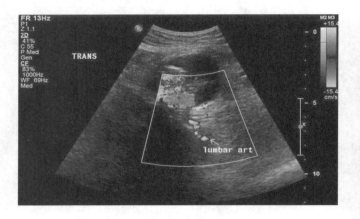 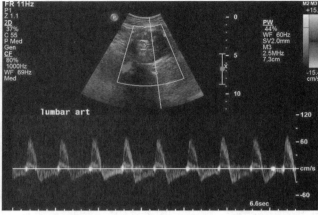

CASE STUDY

Review the information and answer the following questions.

1. A 64-year-old male presents with a pulsatile abdominal mass. The patient has a history of hypertension and smoking. The images were taken during his duplex ultrasound evaluation. What is demonstrated in this patient? Are the ultrasound findings consistent with the patient's clinical presentation?

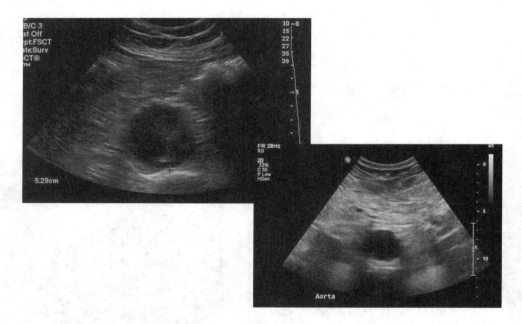

2. A 67-year-old male presents to the vascular lab for follow-up following recent endovascular stent graft repair of his AAA. Upon questioning, the patient states that he has noticed pain and a pulsatile mass in his left groin. What is the likely cause of the pain and pulsatility in this patient's groin? What documentation should be recorded during this patient's duplex ultrasound evaluation?

The Mesenteric Arteries

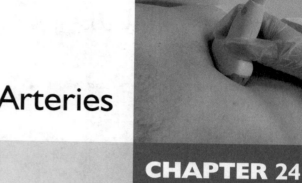

REVIEW OF GLOSSARY TERMS

Matching

Match the key terms with their definitions.

KEY TERMS

1. _____ splanchnic

2. _____ visceral

3. _____ postprandial

4. _____ mesenteric ischemia

5. _____ collateral flow

DEFINITION

a. Occurring after a meal
b. Relating to or affecting the viscera
c. Lack of blood flow to the viscera
d. Relating to additional blood vessels that aid or add to circulation
e. Relating to internal organs or blood vessels in the abdominal cavity

ANATOMY AND PHYSIOLOGY REVIEW

Image Labeling

Complete the labels in the images that follow.

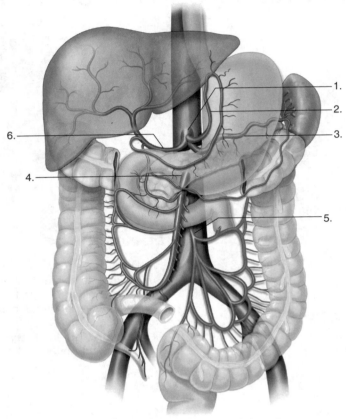

1. The abdominal aorta and mesenteric branches.

CHAPTER REVIEW

Multiple Choice

Complete each question by circling the best answer.

1. What is the first major branch arising from the abdominal aorta?
   a. superior mesenteric artery
   b. celiac artery
   c. inferior mesenteric artery
   d. right renal artery

2. What is the most common indication for mesenteric artery duplex evaluation?
   a. acute mesenteric ischemia
   b. median arcuate ligament compression syndrome
   c. chronic mesenteric ischemia
   d. mesenteric artery aneurysms

3. How many mesenteric arteries are typically involved in atherosclerotic occlusive disease before a patient becomes symptomatic?
   a. 1
   b. 2
   c. 3
   d. 4

4. When does the abdominal pain many patients feel, which is associated with chronic mesenteric ischemia, typically occur?
   a. after eating
   b. in a fasting state
   c. constantly (fasting and nonfasting)
   d. with aerobic exercise

5. Because of the abdominal pain, which of the following do patients often experience?

   a. overeating and weight gain

   b. fear of exercise

   c. nausea and vomiting

   d. fear of food and weight loss

6. Which of the following is a collateral system that is present in the mesenteric vascular system?

   a. pancreaticoduodenal arcade

   b. arc of Riolan

   c. internal iliac to inferior mesenteric artery connections

   d. all the above

7. From which vessel does a replaced right hepatic artery originate most often?

   a. celiac artery

   b. superior mesenteric artery

   c. right renal artery

   d. inferior mesenteric artery

8. With a patient in a fasting state, what should the superior mesenteric artery exhibit?

   a. high-resistance flow pattern

   b. low-resistance flow pattern

   c. mixed high- and low-resistance flow pattern

   d. respiratory phasic flow pattern

9. Standard criteria for determining velocity thresholds for identifying stenosis in the celiac and superior mesenteric arteries were determined with the patient in what state?

   a. fasting

   b. postprandial

   c. upright

   d. pre- and postprandial

10. Which of the following vessels does the term "seagull sign" describe?

    a. superior mesenteric artery and its major branches

    b. inferior mesenteric artery and its major branches

    c. celiac, hepatic, and splenic arteries

    d. left and right renal arteries

11. What should Doppler waveforms obtained from the celiac, splenic, and hepatic arteries demonstrate?

    a. high-resistance flow

    b. mixed high- and low-resistance flow

    c. prolonged systolic upstrokes

    d. low-resistance flow

12. During a mesenteric artery evaluation, retrograde flow is noted in the common hepatic artery. What does this finding suggest?

    a. common hepatic artery stenosis

    b. celiac artery occlusion

    c. superior mesenteric artery stenosis

    d. replaced right hepatic artery

13. Which technique can NOT be used to positively identify and differentiate the celiac and superior mesenteric vessels?

    a. Having the patient suspend breathing to reduce vessel movement.

    b. Visualizing both the celiac and superior mesenteric arteries in the same image.

    c. Visualizing aliasing with color flow in the superior mesenteric artery.

    d. Documenting characteristic low-resistance flow in the celiac artery.

14. What can turning color-flow imaging off help identify?

    a. arterial dissection

    b. characterization of atherosclerotic plaque

    c. stent placement within the vessel

    d. all the above

15. During duplex evaluation of the mesenteric vessels, the SMA is noted to have velocities of 350 cm/s proximally with velocities of close to 300 cm/s in the mid-segment. No spectral broadening or turbulence is noted. With which of the following are these findings consistent?

    a. compensatory flow through the SMA likely caused by occlusion of the celiac artery

    b. significant stenosis of the SMA through its proximal and mid-segments

    c. occlusion of the SMA with reconstitution in the mid-segment

    d. normal SMA findings with normal velocities

16. Which of the following describes the velocity criteria for diagnosis of >70% in the celiac and superior mesenteric arteries?

    a. >275 cm/s PSV in the celiac and >200 cm/s PSV in the superior mesenteric artery

    b. >325 cm/s PSV in both the celiac and superior mesenteric arteries

    c. >200 cm/s PSV in the celiac and >275 cm/s PSV in the superior mesenteric artery

    d. >50 cm/s EDV in the celiac and >55 cm/s EDV in the superior mesenteric artery

17. Why may standard duplex ultrasound velocity criteria for mesenteric vessels NOT be accurate after treatment by stent placement?

    a. Velocities in treated vessels are considerably lower than standard criteria.

    b. Velocities in treated vessels are typically higher than standard criteria.

    c. Stented vessels are not well visualized on duplex scanning.

    d. Stent struts artifactually decrease reflections, making Doppler signals inaccurate.

18. What is transient compression of the celiac artery origin during exhalation, which is relieved by inhalation?

    a. acute mesenteric ischemia

    b. atherosclerotic disease at the celiac artery origin

    c. compression of celiac artery from abdominal aortic aneurysm

    d. median arcuate ligament compression syndrome

19. Visceral artery aneurysms are rare; however, the greatest incidence of aneurysms occurs in which of the following vessels?

    a. splenic artery

    b. common hepatic artery

    c. celiac artery

    d. superior mesenteric artery

20. What is the general role of the vascular laboratory in the diagnosis of acute mesenteric ischemia?

    a. Identification of the thrombus at the origin of the SMA.

    b. No role due to the emergent nature of the illness.

    c. Characterization of the stenosis and degree of narrowing.

    d. Identification of the branch vessel in which embolus is likely to have occurred.

Fill-in-the-Blank

1. The celiac artery is best visualized with the transducer oriented in a _____ plane, whereas the superior mesenteric artery is best visualized with the transducer oriented in a _____ plane.

2. The diagnosis of chronic mesenteric ischemia is often _____ because the disorder is rare and the symptoms may be due to a vast number of abdominal disorders.

3. Postprandial abdominal pain that occurs when there is insufficient visceral blood flow to support the increased oxygen demand required by intestinal motility, secretion, and absorption is often termed _____.

4. The inferior mesenteric artery arises from the aorta just proximal to the _____.

5. A replaced right hepatic artery originating from the superior mesenteric artery should be suspected when the SMA demonstrates a _____ flow pattern.

6. It is critically important for the patient to fast for at least 6 hours prior to mesenteric artery evaluation because the superior mesenteric artery changes dramatically from _____ resistance to _____ resistance after eating.

7. When performing spectral Doppler and high velocities are noted in a mesenteric artery, it is important to document _____ to confirm a flow-limiting stenosis.

8. The term "seagull sign" refers to the sonographic appearance of the _____ artery and its branches, the _____ and _____ arteries.

9. The celiac artery and its branches typically display and _____-resistance flow pattern, whereas the superior and inferior mesenteric arteries demonstrate a _____-flow pattern.

10. A technique that can be used to decrease movement of mesenteric vessels and help capture Doppler waveforms with a correct angle is to have the patient _____.

11. In the presence of celiac artery occlusion, the common hepatic artery almost always demonstrates _____ flow.

12. An important technique to use when evaluating the mesenteric vessels that can help detect vessel wall abnormalities or vessel tortuosity is to inspect the image with _____ imaging only.

13. In preparation for a duplex scan after mesenteric revascularization, the _____ note will detail the location of the proximal and distal anastomoses and type of graft or other intervention.

14. When following-up on a mesenteric bypass graft, if the PSV is >300 or <50 cm/s, it is recommended to _____ the time between surveillance scans.

15. Increased velocities in the absence of stenosis could be the result of _____ flow.

16. According to one study, a PSV in the celiac artery of >200 cm/s and a PSV in the SMA of >275 cm/s corresponded to a stenosis of _____%

17. According to one study, when end-diastolic velocities are used as thresholds for >50% stenosis the corresponding velocities are _____ cm/s in the celiac artery and _____ cm/s in the superior mesenteric artery.

18. Recent studies suggest velocity guidelines for IMA stenosis, with a PSV of _____ corresponding to a >50% stenosis.

19. Percutaneous visceral artery intervention has lower morbidity/mortality rates than traditional surgical repair; however, it is associated with higher _____ rates and the requirement for re-intervention.

20. An advantage of using duplex ultrasound to evaluate median arcuate ligament compression syndrome is that Doppler waveforms can be obtained during changes in _____.

21. Splenic artery aneurysm, when discovered during pregnancy, is associated with a 95% _____ rate, leading to high maternal and fetal mortality.

22. Visceral artery dissections are most common in the _____ and are often extensions of aortic dissection.

23. In patients with suspected MALS, if velocities fail to normalize with inspiration, the patient can be put in a _____ position.

24. Embolus to or thrombosis of the mesenteric arteries can lead to _____.

25. Symptoms associated with the abovementioned pathology are typically described as pain _____ to physical findings.

Short Answer

1. What is the typical patient presentation of chronic mesenteric ischemia?

2. What is the purpose of using a "test meal" when evaluating the mesenteric vessels?

3. How can compensatory flow be distinguished from elevated velocities due to stenosis?

IMAGE EVALUATION/PATHOLOGY

Review the images and answer the following questions.

1. A 32-year-old female presents to the vascular lab for an abdominal bruit. These images were taken during the exam of the abdominal aorta. What is present in these images?

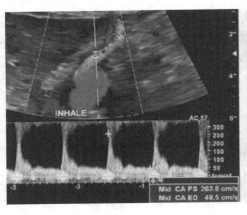 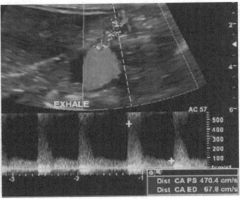

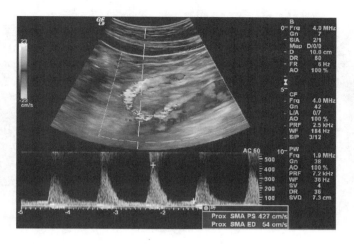

2. A 73-year-old female presents to the vascular lab with abdominal pain after eating and a recent history of weight loss. Duplex imaging of the abdominal aorta and its branches reveals this image. What is demonstrated in this image? What other vessels should be evaluated and why?

CASE STUDY

Review the information and answer the following questions.

1. A 68-year-old female presents to the emergency department with acute onset of severe abdominal pain. Upon physical examination, nothing is found to be consistent with the amount of pain the patient is in. Based on this limited history, what should be suspected? What imaging examinations should the patient undergo?

2. A 40-year-old multiparous female presents for abdominal duplex examination for suspicion of gallbladder disease. During this evaluation, an anechoic, circular mass is noted superior to the pancreas that appears to be in communication with the splenic artery. Color and spectral Doppler demonstrate flow within the mass. What should be suspected in this patient? What is the prognosis for this patient?

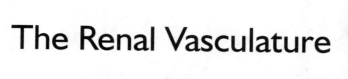

The Renal Vasculature

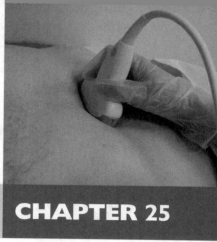

REVIEW OF GLOSSARY TERMS

Matching

Match the key terms with their definitions.

KEY TERMS

1. _____ renal–aortic velocity ratio

2. _____ poststenotic signal

3. _____ renal medulla

4. _____ renal hilum

5. _____ renal ostium

6. _____ renal sinus

7. _____ renal cortex

8. _____ renal parenchymal disease

9. _____ renal artery stenosis

10. _____ renal artery stent

11. _____ suprasternal notch

12. _____ symphysis pubis/pubic bone

DEFINITION

a. The central echogenic cavity of the kidney; contains the renal artery, renal vein, and collecting and lymphatic systems

b. Narrowing of the renal artery, most commonly as a result of atherosclerotic disease or medial fibromuscular dysplasia

c. The visible indentation at the base of the neck where the neck joins the sternum

d. A medical disorder affecting the tissue function of the kidneys

e. The peak systolic renal artery velocity divided by the peak systolic aortic velocity recorded at the level of the celiac and/or superior mesenteric arteries; used to identify flow-limiting renal artery stenosis

f. The area through which the renal artery, vein, and ureter enter the kidney

g. A tiny tube inserted into a stenotic renal artery at the time of arterial dilation; usually metallic mesh in structure; holds the artery open

h. The prominence of the pelvic bones noted in the lower abdomen

i. A Doppler spectral waveform recorded immediately distal to a flow-reducing stenosis that exhibits decreased peak systolic velocity and disordered flow

j. The opening of the renal artery from the aortic wall

k. The middle area of the kidney lying between the sinus and the cortex; contains renal pyramids

l. The outermost area of the kidney tissue lying just beneath the renal capsule

ANATOMY AND PHYSIOLOGY REVIEW

Image Labeling

Complete the labels in the images that follow.

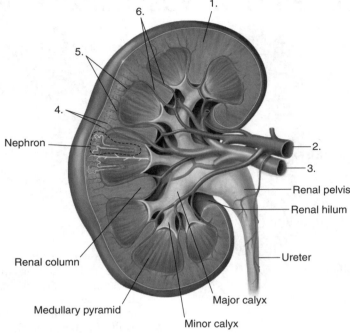

1. Diagram illustrating the vasculature of the kidneys.

CHAPTER REVIEW

Multiple Choice

Complete each question by circling the best answer.

1. It is estimated that up to how many hypertensive patients have underlying renal artery disease?
   a. 50%
   b. 40%
   c. 6%
   d. 15%

2. Which of the following is NOT a limitation of contrast angiography?
   a. detailed anatomic information
   b. lack of hemodynamic information
   c. no identification of functional significance of renal artery disease
   d. invasive with possible nephrotoxic contrast

3. Which of the following is true regarding duplex ultrasound assessment of the renal vasculature?
   a. provides anatomic information
   b. provides hemodynamic information
   c. painless and noninvasive
   d. all the above

4. What is the normal length measurement of the kidney?
   a. 4 to 5 cm
   b. 8 to 13 cm
   c. 10 to 15 cm
   d. 5 to 7 cm

5. What are kidneys that are joined at the lower poles by an isthmus of tissue which lies anterior to the aorta?
   a. ectopic kidneys
   b. cross-fused kidneys
   c. horseshoe kidneys
   d. junctional kidneys

6. Why is the renal sinus normally brightly echogenic on a sonographic image?
   a. lymphatic vessel location
   b. fat and fibrous tissue in the sinus
   c. increased blood flow in the area
   d. fluid from the collecting system

7. What are the triangular-shaped structures within the inner portion of the kidney that carry urine from the cortex to the renal pelvis?
   a. nephrons
   b. columns of Bertin
   c. renal pyramids
   d. renal calyces

8. The right renal artery initially courses _____ from the aorta, then passes _____ to the inferior vena cava.
   a. posterolateral, anterior
   b. posterior, superior
   c. anterolateral, lateral
   d. anterolateral, posterior

9. Which vessel courses anterior to the aorta but posterior to the superior mesenteric artery and anterior to both renal arteries?
   a. splenic vein
   b. right renal vein
   c. left renal vein
   d. inferior mesenteric vein

10. In which of the following renal artery segments does atherosclerotic disease in the renal artery typically occur?
    a. origin to proximal third
    b. distal renal artery just before entering the kidney
    c. mid-to-distal segment
    d. interlobar arteries within the renal parenchyma

11. Which of the following patients would be suspected of fibromuscular dysplasia in the renal artery?
    a. an 85-year-old diabetic male
    b. a 66-year-old female with a history of well-controlled hypertension and smoking
    c. a 25-year-old male with chronic asthma
    d. a 32-year-old female with poorly controlled hypertension

12. What is the most appropriate transducer for use in the evaluation of the renal arteries?
    a. 7 to 10 MHz straight linear
    b. 2 to 5 MHz curved linear
    c. 1 to 2 MHz vector array
    d. 5 to 8 MHz phased sector array

13. At which level is a spectral Doppler waveform with peak systolic velocity needed from the aorta for use in the renal–aortic ratio?
    a. proximal, at the level of the celiac and superior mesenteric arteries
    b. mid, at the level of the renal arteries
    c. distal, at the level of the inferior mesenteric artery
    d. distal, at the level of the common iliac bifurcation

14. To identify the renal artery ostia from a midline approach, an image is obtained from which location?
    a. transverse, at the level of the celiac artery
    b. sagittal, at the level of the celiac artery
    c. transverse, slightly inferior to the superior mesenteric artery
    d. sagittal, slightly superior to the left renal vein

15. Which of the following is an ultrasound modality that has a low-angle dependence that may be helpful in identifying duplicate renal arteries?
    a. color-flow Doppler
    b. power Doppler
    c. spectral Doppler
    d. pulse inversion Doppler

16. Using which angle of insonation are flow patterns within the kidney parenchyma typically obtained with a spectral Doppler?
    a. 60 degrees
    b. 90 degrees
    c. 0 degrees
    d. 45 degrees

17. When comparing renal length from side to side, how much of a difference suggests compromised flow in the smaller kidney?
    a. 1 cm
    b. 2 mm
    c. 3 mm
    d. 3 cm

18. Which of the following describe normal spectral Doppler waveform characteristics in the renal artery?
    a. high-resistance, minimal diastolic flow with velocities in the range of 90 to 120 cm/s
    b. low-resistance, high-diastolic flow with velocities in the range of 90 to 120 cm/s
    c. low-resistance, minimal diastolic flow with velocities in the range of 10 to 120 cm/s
    d. high-resistance, high-diastolic flow with velocities in the range of 50 to 70 cm/s

19. A patient presents to the vascular laboratory for a renal artery duplex evaluation. During the examination, velocities in the right renal artery origin reach 175 cm/s with no evidence of poststenotic turbulence. Velocities on the left were 100 cm/s. What do these findings suggest?
    a. right renal artery stenosis <60%
    b. left renal artery stenosis <60%
    c. right renal artery stenosis >60%
    d. left renal artery stenosis >60%

20. Which of the following spectral Doppler waveform changes will NOT occur distal to a hemodynamically significant stenosis of the renal artery?
    a. delayed systolic upstroke
    b. loss of compliance peak
    c. decreased peak systolic velocity
    d. increased peak systolic velocity

21. Which of the following findings within the kidney are consistent with renal artery occlusion?
    a. kidney length of >10 cm, velocities less than 10 cm/s in the renal cortex
    b. kidney length of <9 cm, velocities less than 10 cm/s in the renal cortex
    c. kidney length >13 cm with no detectable flow within the renal parenchyma
    d. kidney length <9 cm, velocities greater than 20 cm/s in the renal cortex

22. A patient presents to the vascular lab with suspected acute tubular necrosis. Which of the following findings on the renal artery duplex exam would be consistent with this condition?
    a. renal artery velocities >180 cm/s, EDR of 0.35
    b. renal artery velocities >180 cm/s, RI of 0.6
    c. renal artery velocities of 70 cm/s, EDR of 0.19
    d. renal artery velocities of 70 cm/s, RI of 0.5

23. What is measured to determine acceleration time?
    a. onset of systole to the early systolic peak
    b. onset of systole to the end of diastole
    c. onset of diastole to the early systolic peak
    d. end diastole to end systole

24. During a renal artery duplex exam, proximal aortic velocities of 100 cm/s, proximal right renal artery velocity of 200 cm/s, and proximal left renal artery velocities of 400 cm/s were found. Which of the following describes these findings?
    a. right RAR = 2.0, <60% stenosis; left RAR = 0.4, <60% stenosis
    b. right RAR = 0.2, >60% stenosis, left RAR = 0.4, >60% stenosis
    c. right RAR = 2.0, <60% stenosis; left RAR = 4.0, >60% stenosis
    d. right RAR = 0.2, >60% stenosis; left RAR = 4.0, <60% stenosis

25. During the renal artery duplex exam, in the above question for which renal artery would you expect to see poststenotic turbulence?
    a. right
    b. left
    c. both
    d. neither

26. Which of the following may result in misinterpretation of the hilar acceleration time?
    a. elevated renovascular resistance
    b. systemic arterial stiffness
    c. renal artery stenosis in the 60% to 79% range
    d. all the above

27. Under which conditions is the renal to aortic ratio likely inaccurate?
    a. The abdominal aortic velocities are between 75 and 90 cm/s.
    b. The abdominal aortic velocities are over 100 cm/s or below 40 cm/s.
    c. The renal artery velocities exceed 300 cm/s.
    d. The renal artery velocities are below 100 cm/s.

28. During renal duplex evaluation, the left renal vein near the hilum is noted to have continuous, nonphasic low-velocity flow. What do these findings suggest?
    a. renal artery stenosis
    b. normal renal vein findings
    c. proximal renal vein thrombosis
    d. distal renal vein thrombosis

29. A patient presents to the vascular lab for follow-up after renal artery stent placement. Velocities within the distal segment of the stent reach 250 cm/s. At other follow-ups at 6 and 12 months, velocities in the distal stent remain 250 cm/s. What are these findings consistent with?
    a. increased velocity because of size mismatch from the stent to native vessel
    b. fixed stenosis at the distal end of the stent
    c. kinking of the stent, creating artificially elevated velocities
    d. stent collapse and failure

30. Which of the following represents renal duplex findings that demonstrate a high risk for renal atrophy and likely unsuccessful renal revascularization?
    a. renal artery PSV <400 cm/s and cortical EDV >10 cm/s
    b. renal artery PSV >400 cm/s and cortical EDV <5 cm/s
    c. renal artery PSV >160 cm/s and cortical EDV <10 cm/s
    d. renal artery PSV >200 cm/s and cortical EDV <5 cm/s

Fill-in-the-Blank

1. Patients with sudden onset of chronic hypertension, azotemia, unexplained renal insufficiency, or pulmonary edema should be evaluated for _____.

2. In most patients, renal artery disease is correctable with treatment providing _____ for hypertension and stabilization of renal function in patients with chronic renal failure.

3. Because of the _____ of the contrast agents, computed tomography angiography is often reserved for use as secondary confirmatory study.

4. The kidneys are located _____ in the dorsal abdominal cavity between the 12th thoracic and third lumbar vertebrae.

5. For the purpose of sonographic examination of the kidney, it is divided into _____ main areas.

6. The renal arteries can be identified approximately _____ cm below the _____ plane, with the left renal artery slightly more cephalad than the right.

7. Duplicate main renal arteries which enter the kidney through the renal hilum or accessory polar arteries are present in _____% of patients.

8. Owing to the location of the inferior vena cava, the right renal vein has a _____ course, and the left renal vein typically courses _____ to the aorta.

9. The second most common curable cause of renovascular disease is _____, which occurs most commonly in women aged 25 to 50 years.

10. Elevating the examination table, keeping the patient close to the sonographer's side, and not overextending the arm are all ways to maintain _____ positioning.

11. Extrinsic compression of the left renal vein may result in _____ syndrome.

12. From a midline abdominal approach, the Doppler sample volume can be walked from the _____ lumen through the _____ to detect abnormal flow patterns.

13. A useful approach to identify the ostia of the renal arteries that involves having the patient in a decubitus position and imaging the aorta in a longitudinal plane to view the renal arteries from the lateral aortic walls is termed the _____ approach.

14. _____ Doppler is valuable in identifying these duplicate renal arteries because of its lower angle dependence and sensitivity to low-flow states.

15. An alternate position to access the distal segments of the renal arteries in the _____ position, with the patient's midsection flexed over a pillow.

16. In addition to evaluation of the renal vasculature, the _____ should be examined for cortical thinning, renal calculi, masses, cysts, or hydronephrosis.

17. Accuracy of renal length is enhanced by averaging _____ separate measurements.

18. In the presence of renal vein _____, renal artery waveforms demonstrate retrograde, blunted diastolic flow components.

19. Improved diagnostic accuracy has been shown in the liver, mesenteric, and peripheral vessels with the use of _____.

20. The proximal aorta demonstrates rapid systolic upstroke and _____ flow during diastole, whereas the distal abdominal aorta demonstrates a _____ flow pattern that reflects the elevated vascular resistance of the lower extremities.

21. An early _____ peak is often seen on the upstroke to systole in a normal renal artery.

22. When the degree of renal artery narrowing exceeds _____%, the systolic upstroke is delayed, the compliance peak is lost, and the PSV will decrease distally.

23. With chronic renal artery occlusion, the PSV in the cortex will be less than _____ cm/s, and pole-to-pole length of the kidney will be less than _____ cm.

24. When parenchymal disease is present, increased renovascular _____ is demonstrated throughout the kidney, characterized by _____ diastolic flow.

25. Indirect renal hilar evaluations use _____ index or time to provide assessment of renal artery stenosis.

26. Current diagnostic criteria for identification of renal artery stenosis are based on the _____ ratio greater than _____.

27. Continuous, nonphasic low-velocity flow is noted in the renal vein in the presence of _____.

28. When evaluating a stented renal artery, velocity _____ are typically identified, making identification of restenosis difficult.

29. Revascularization is often unsuccessful in kidneys with a pole-to-pole length less than _____.

30. The most common cause of renal artery stenosis in the pediatric patient is _____.

Short Answer

1. Atherosclerotic stenosis and fibromuscular dysplasia are the most commonly observed renal artery pathologies. What are the other complications that should be considered during sonographic examination of the renal vascular system?

2. Describe the appropriate patient preparation and positioning for a renal artery duplex examination.

3. List the diagnostic criteria used to determine renal artery stenosis and intrinsic renal parenchymal disease.

4. What are the limitations of indirect renal hilar examination?

5. While the scanning technique does not differ between adult and pediatric patient, what differences should the vascular sonographer be aware of between adult and pediatric patients when assessing renal arteries and kidneys?

IMAGE EVALUATION/PATHOLOGY

Review the images and answer the following questions.

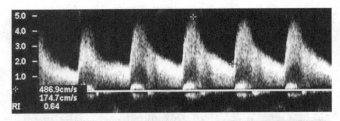

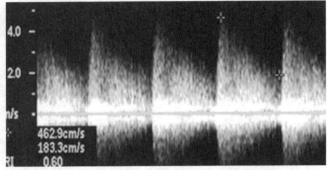

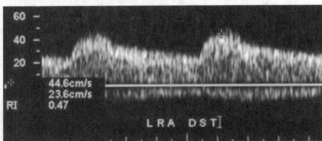

1. These spectral Doppler waveforms were taken from the left renal artery origin, proximal, and distal segments, respectively. What do these images suggest?

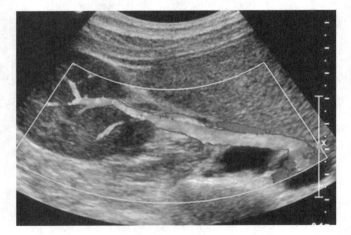

2. This image demonstrates the right renal artery and inferior vena cava. What anomaly is present?

CASE STUDY

Review the information and answer the following questions.

1. A 68-year-old male with chronic hypertension presents to the vascular laboratory for renal artery duplex evaluation. The patient's history also includes diabetes, hyperlipidemia, angina, and smoking. During the renal artery duplex exam, the following was found: right renal artery PSV 325 cm/s and EDV 140 cm/s with turbulence noted just past the origin; left renal artery of 185 cm/s and EDV 80 cm/s, no turbulence is noted; proximal aorta PSV 85 cm/s. In the renal hila, acceleration times are 105 ms on the right and 80 ms on the left. What do these findings suggest?

2. A 37-year-old female presents to the vascular lab with uncontrolled hypertension for renal artery duplex examination. What disease process should be suspected in this patient? What should the vascular technologist be on the lookout for during a renal artery duplex examination?

3. An 82-year-old female presents to the vascular laboratory with elevated serum creatinine and blood urea nitrogen levels. During renal artery duplex examination, velocities from the renal arteries remain within normal limits. Upon evaluation of the renal parenchyma, peak systolic velocities are 25 cm/s with end-diastolic velocities of 6 cm/s, bilaterally. What is the resistive index and diastolic to systolic ratio in the kidneys? What do these findings suggest?

The Inferior Vena Cava and Iliac Veins

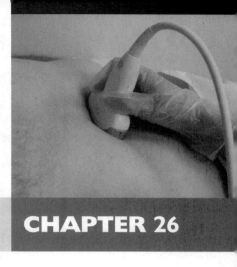

REVIEW OF GLOSSARY TERMS

Matching

Match the key terms with their definitions.

KEY TERMS

1. _____ retroperitoneum

2. _____ inferior vena cava filter

3. _____ pulmonary embolus

4. _____ thrombosis

5. _____ confluence

DEFINITION

a. The obstruction of the pulmonary arteries, usually from detached fragments of a blood clot that travels from the lower extremity

b. The union of two or more veins to form a larger vein; the equivalent of a bifurcation in the arterial system

c. The space between the abdominal cavity and the muscles and bones of the posterior abdominal wall

d. Partial or complete occlusion of a blood vessel due to clot

e. A typically cone-shaped medical device designed to prevent pulmonary embolism

ANATOMY AND PHYSIOLOGY REVIEW

Image Labeling

Complete the labels in the image that follows.

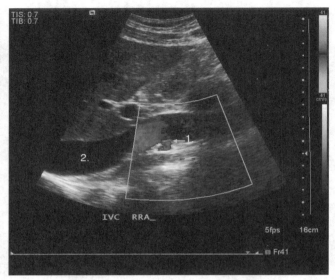

1. Sagittal image through the mid-abdomen.

CHAPTER REVIEW

Multiple Choice

Complete each question by circling the best answer.

1. Which of the following vessels extends as the external iliac vein?
   a. common iliac vein
   b. great saphenous vein
   c. common femoral vein
   d. inferior vena cava

2. In well-hydrated patients, what is the mean diameter of the inferior vena cava at the level of the renal veins?
   a. 17 to 20 mm
   b. 10 to 15 mm
   c. 2 to 3 cm
   d. 3 to 5 cm

3. Where does the left-sided IVC in a duplicate system typically terminate?
   a. splenic vein
   b. right renal vein
   c. superior mesenteric vein
   d. left renal vein

4. Upon ultrasound examination, the hepatic veins are noted to drain directly into the right atrium. What does this finding suggest?
   a. normal findings in the hepatic veins
   b. congenital absence of the inferior vena cava
   c. membranous obstruction of the intrahepatic IVC
   d. duplicate inferior vena cava syndrome

5. Which of the following is an impediment to visualizing the inferior vena cava?
   a. overlying bowel gas
   b. morbid obesity
   c. open abdominal wounds
   d. all the above

6. While applying pressure to the patient's abdomen may disperse bowel gas to make visualization of the IVC easier, why must care be taken?
   a. Excessive force can compress the IVC.
   b. Gentle pressure may result in bruising of the patient.
   c. Excessive force may result in compression of the aorta.
   d. Gentle pressure can create a stenosis in the IVC.

7. On what signs and symptoms should the history and physical examination related to the inferior vena cava and iliac veins focus?
   a. tumor infiltration and cancer risk
   b. venous thrombosis and insufficiency
   c. liver function and cirrhosis
   d. claudication and atherosclerotic risk factors

8. From a coronal plane in the left lateral decubitus position, what landmark can be used to identify the confluence of the common iliac veins to create the IVC?
   a. superior pole of the right kidney
   b. left lobe of the liver
   c. inferior pole of the right kidney
   d. inferior pole of the left kidney

9. Which of the following describes normal IVC and iliac vein imaging characteristics?
   a. thin, echogenic walls with anechoic lumens
   b. thin, hypoechoic walls with hyperechoic lumens
   c. thick, muscular walls that are hypoechoic with hyperechoic lumens
   d. anechoic walls with hypoechoic lumens

10. What is the most common pathologic finding in the IVC and iliac veins?
    a. tumor extension from renal cell carcinoma
    b. thrombus extension from deep venous thrombosis in the legs
    c. isolated thrombosis of the IVC
    d. venous dissection through the iliac veins

11. Newly formed thrombus appears virtually _____, whereas more advanced thrombus appears _____.
    a. hyperechoic, anechoic
    b. hyperechoic, hypoechoic
    c. hypoechoic, hypoechoic
    d. anechoic, hyperechoic

12. From what do intraluminal tumors in the inferior vena cava most commonly arise?
    a. pancreatic carcinoma
    b. colon carcinoma
    c. renal cell carcinoma
    d. bladder carcinoma

13. How can intraluminal tumors be distinguished from thrombosis?
    a. Tumors demonstrate flow within the mass.
    b. Tumors demonstrate anechoic texture.
    c. Tumors demonstrate lack of flow in the mass.
    d. Tumors demonstrate change in echogenicity over time.

14. Which Doppler mode would best be able to detect the slow-flow states that are typically seen in the inferior vena cava and iliac veins?
    a. color Doppler
    b. power Doppler
    c. spectral Doppler
    d. CW Doppler

15. In what ways can color-flow Doppler be particularly useful in identifying tissue bruits and pulsatile flow?
    a. filter perforation
    b. deep venous thrombosis
    c. tumor extension
    d. aortocaval fistula

16. During spectral Doppler analysis of the iliac system, continuous flow is noted in the common iliac veins bilaterally. What does this finding suggest?
    a. obstruction in the common iliac veins
    b. obstruction in the common femoral veins
    c. obstruction in the inferior vena cava
    d. normal findings in the common iliac veins

17. What is the condition that occurs when the left common iliac vein is compressed between the overlying right common iliac artery and underlying vertebral body?
    a. May–Thurner's syndrome
    b. Raynaud's syndrome
    c. arcuate ligament syndrome
    d. Paget–Schroetter's syndrome

18. What is filter placement in the inferior vena cava designed to prevent?
    a. thrombus extension from the lower extremities
    b. pulmonary embolus
    c. thrombus extension from the intrahepatic inferior vena cava
    d. tumor extension from the renal veins

19. Which of the following is a dependable marker for ultrasound identification of the level of the renal veins for IVC filter placement?
    a. superior mesenteric artery
    b. superior mesenteric vein
    c. left renal vein
    d. right renal artery

20. On sonographic evaluation, which of the following describes the appearance of an IVC filter?
    a. hypoechoic, circular rings within the IVC lumen
    b. hyperechoic, circular rings within the IVC lumen
    c. echogenic lines that converge to a point
    d. hypoechoic lines that converge to a point

Fill-in-the-Blank

1. The pelvic viscera and musculature are drained by the _____ veins.

2. Patients with congestive heart failure may present with _____ or excessively large IVC diameter.

3. The presence of a fibrous septum in the IVC just cephalad to the insertion of the right hepatic vein would indicate _____ of the intrahepatic IVC.

4. When evaluating the IVC, the height of the bed should be adjusted so that the level of the patient's _____ is slightly lower than the sonographer's _____ to ergonomically apply pressure.

5. The inferior vena cava will appear oval shaped when viewed in a(n) _____ plane.

6. Landmarks that can be used to identify the IVC in a longitudinal plane include the _____, which lies to the left of the IVC and the _____, which lies anterior to the IVC.

7. The _____ plane may offer better imaging of the distal IVC and confluence of the common iliac veins.

8. When evaluating the iliac veins, the patient should be positioned supine with the bed in a(n) _____ position.

9. With quiet respiration, the _____ of the IVC may appear to change with the phasic changes in abdominal pressure.

10. Acute thrombus may appear virtually anechoic on grayscale; therefore, _____ is/are important to the examination.

11. Thrombus that does not completely obstruct flow may be detected by grayscale imaging demonstrating _____ echogenic material in the IVC or iliac vein.

12. Intraluminal tumors may completely or partially obstruct the IVC or iliac veins, resulting in _____ collateral veins and _____ of the distal IVC and iliac veins.

13. An IVC filter is typically placed just _____ to the renal veins.

14. Echogenic material found within and around an IVC filter represents trapped _____ and should be considered an abnormal finding.

15. In an ultrasound evaluation of the IVC with filter placement, visualization of a hematoma adjacent to the IVC likely indicates _____.

16. Normally, the proximal IVC demonstrates a _____ waveform pattern, whereas the distal IVC and iliac veins demonstrate respiratory _____.

17. Unlike in the lower extremity veins, the iliac veins cannot be evaluated with transducer _____ maneuvers; therefore, spectral Doppler becomes important in detecting iliac vein thrombosis.

18. Cardiac pulsations detected in the iliac veins is often a sign of _____.

19. Loss of respiratory phasicity and inability to augment the signal with distal thigh compression in an iliac vein indicate _____.

20. The condition that occurs when the left common iliac vein is compressed between the overlying right common iliac artery and commonly presents as left iliac vein DVT is _____.

21. When using duplex ultrasound for guidance for IVC filter placement, the _____ can be used as a marker to determine the correct level for filter placement.

22. When guiding filter placement, flushing saline through the initial sheath creates _____ at the tip which can aid in identification.

23. Benefits of ultrasound guidance for filter placement include performance of the procedure at the bedside and lack of exposure to _____.

24. Color imaging with IVUS can help differentiate the _____ lumen from the _____.

25. IVUS has excellent sensitivity in detecting _____ vein segments and in the placement of iliac vein stents.

Short Answer

1. What are the tributaries that drain into the inferior vena cava?

2. What Doppler findings are consistent with iliac vein compression syndrome?

3. What can IVUS be used to detect in the IVC and iliac vein system?

IMAGE EVALUATION/PATHOLOGY

Review the images and answer the following questions.

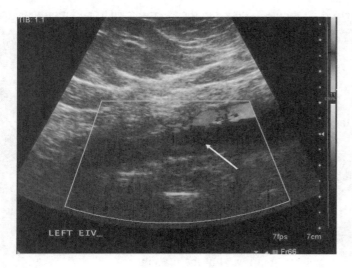

1. Describe the findings in this image. What additional information would aid in the diagnosis?

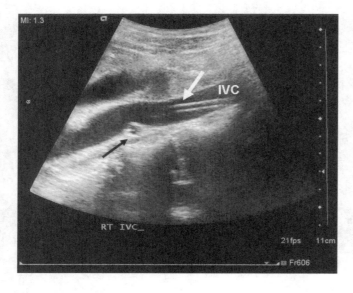

2. What is demonstrated in this image, indicated by the white arrow? What is its purpose?

3. What is the black arrow pointing to, and why is this structure important?

CASE STUDY

Review the information and answer the following questions.

1. A 57-year-old female presents with bilateral lower extremity swelling. The patient has a history of renal cell carcinoma. What should the vascular technologist be concerned about in this patient?

2. During inferior vena cava and iliac vein ultrasound evaluation, a thrombus is noted in the right external iliac vein. Describe the spectral Doppler findings in the following vessels, including responses to distal augmentation maneuvers.

   a. Right common femoral vein

   b. Right common iliac vein

   c. Inferior vena cava

   d. Left common iliac vein

The Hepatoportal System

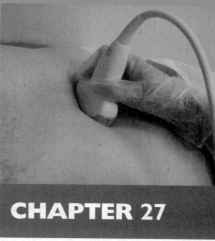

CHAPTER 27

REVIEW OF GLOSSARY TERMS

Matching

Match the key terms with their definitions.

KEY TERMS

1. _____ hepatopetal

2. _____ hepatofugal

3. _____ portal hypertension

4. _____ Budd–Chiari syndrome

5. _____ ascites

6. _____ helical portal vein flow

7. _____ hepatic arterial buffer response (HABR)

8. _____ hepatic hydrothorax

9. _____ transjugular intrahepatic portosystemic shunt (TIPS)

10. _____ portosystemic collaterals

11. _____ sinusoidal obstruction syndrome (SOS)

DEFINITION

a. An abnormal accumulation of fluid within the peritoneal cavity; most common complication of cirrhosis

b. A percutaneously created connection within the liver between the hepatic vein and portal vein that allows blood flow to bypass the liver as a means to reduce portal pressure in patients with complication related to portal hypertension

c. Elevated pressure gradient between the portal vein and IVC or hepatic veins of 10 to 12 mm Hg or greater

d. Compensatory mechanism to maintain perfusion to the liver by arterial vasodilation when portal vein flow is obstructed in patients with advanced cirrhosis

e. Formation of abnormal blood vessels that shunt portal blood flow bypassing the liver to the systemic circulation, decompressing increased portal venous pressure

f. Hepatic venous outflow obstruction at any level from the small hepatic veins to the junction of the inferior vena cava and the right atrium, regardless of the cause of obstruction

g. A syndrome of tender hepatomegaly, right upper quadrant pain, jaundice, and ascites, most often occurring in patients undergoing hematopoietic cell transplantation, and less commonly following radiation therapy to the live, liver transplantation, and ingestion of alkaloid toxins; formerly known as hepatic veno-occlusive disease

h. Toward the liver, usually referring to normal direction of portal vein flow

i. Spiraling, swirling, "helix" flow pattern demonstrating hepatopetal, hepatofugal, or simultaneous bidirectional flow; uncommon flow pattern seen in 2% of normal patients

j. Away from the liver

k. A pleural effusion in patients with liver cirrhosis in the absence of cardiopulmonary disease; involves passage of ascitic fluid from the peritoneal cavity to the pleural space through diaphragmatic defects

ANATOMY AND PHYSIOLOGY REVIEW

Image Labeling

Complete the labels in the images that follow.

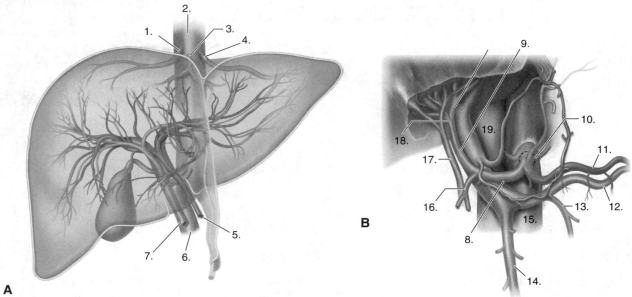

1. Anatomic diagram of the liver.

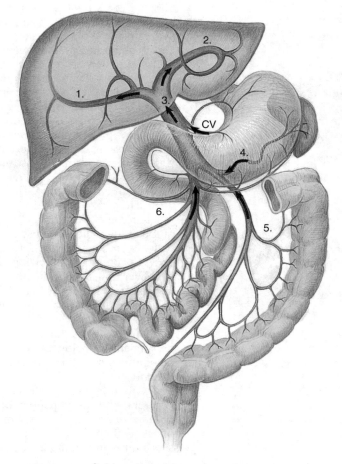

2. Normal portal vascular anatomy.

CHAPTER REVIEW

Multiple Choice

Complete each question by circling the best answer.

1. What percentage of blood is supplied to the liver through the portal vein?
   a. 30%
   b. 50%
   c. 70%
   d. 100%

2. What is the transverse fissure on the visceral surface of the liver between the caudate and quadrate lobes?
   a. main lobar fissure
   b. porta hepatis
   c. ligamentum venosum
   d. falciform ligament

3. Which of the following describes the portal veins within the liver?
   a. thin, invisible walls; course between the liver segments
   b. thin, invisible walls; course within the liver segments
   c. thick, bright walls; course between the liver segments
   d. thick, bright walls; course within the liver segments

4. Which landmark identifies the start of the proper hepatic artery from the common hepatic artery?
   a. gastroduodenal artery
   b. splenic artery
   c. superior mesenteric artery
   d. portal vein

5. Which of the following patient positions offers excellent visualization of the porta hepatis?
   a. transverse epigastric
   b. transverse right costal
   c. right coronal oblique
   d. left coronal oblique

6. At which location should the portal vein diameter be measured?
   a. just inside the liver before it branches into the right and left portal vein
   b. where it crosses the inferior vena cava
   c. at the splenic–superior mesenteric vein confluence
   d. where it crosses the aorta

7. What is normal portal vein diameter with quiet respiration?
   a. ≤13 mm
   b. >16 mm
   c. ≥13 mm
   d. ≤13 cm

8. What does an increase in caliber of less than 20% in the splenic vein during deep inspiration indicate?
   a. splenic vein thrombosis
   b. Budd–Chiari syndrome
   c. portal hypertension
   d. congestive heart failure

9. Which of the following increases blood flow within the portal, splenic, and superior mesenteric veins?
   a. inspiration and ingestion of food
   b. inspiration and exercise
   c. expiration and exercise
   d. expiration and ingestion of food

10. When assessing hepatic vein flow, the S and D waves should show blood flow toward which organ?
    a. liver
    b. heart
    c. spleen
    d. small intestine

11. What is a normal resistive index in the hepatic artery?
    a. 0.2 to 0.4
    b. 0.8 to 1.0
    c. 0.5 to 0.7
    d. 1.3 to 1.5

12. What is the most common etiology for portal hypertension in North America?
    a. portal vein thrombosis
    b. Budd–Chiari syndrome
    c. hepatitis C infection
    d. cirrhosis

13. What is the primary complication of portal hypertension?
    a. portal vein thrombosis
    b. gastrointestinal bleeding
    c. hepatic vein thrombosis
    d. splenomegaly

14. Which of the following is NOT a duplex sonographic finding associated with portal hypertension?
    a. increased portal vein diameter
    b. decreased or absent respiratory variation in portal and splenic veins
    c. hepatopetal flow in the portal and splenic veins
    d. portosystemic collaterals (varices)

15. What is the most common portosystemic collateral shunt in the presence of portal hypertension?
    a. recanalized paraumbilical vein
    b. splenorenal veins
    c. gallbladder varices
    d. coronary–gastroesophageal veins

16. Which of the following is a treatment of portal hypertension that involves jugular vein cannulation with stent placement in the liver?
    a. mesocaval shunt
    b. splenorenal shunt
    c. TIPS
    d. PVTS

17. Which of the following is NOT a normal finding in a transjugular portosystemic shunt?
    a. hepatofugal flow in the main portal vein
    b. velocities within the stent in the range of 90 to 190 cm/s
    c. hepatofugal flow in intrahepatic portal veins beyond the site of stent connection
    d. increased flow velocities in the splenic vein

18. Upon duplex evaluation of the portal system, the vascular technologist visualizes increased portal vein caliber with no detectable flow by color, power, and spectral Doppler. Increased hepatic arterial flow is also documented. What do these findings suggest?
    a. portal hypertension
    b. Budd–Chiari syndrome
    c. cirrhosis
    d. portal vein thrombosis

19. Besides inferior vena cava dilatation, what distinct finding helps differentiate between congestive heart failure and portal hypertension?
    a. increased pulsatility in the portal veins only
    b. increased pulsatility in the hepatic veins only
    c. increased pulsatility in both the portal and hepatic veins
    d. decreased pulsatility in the hepatic veins only

20. Which of the following is NOT a sonographic finding in Budd–Chiari syndrome?
    a. dilatation of the IVC with intraluminal echoes
    b. pulsatile, phasic flow in nonoccluded portions of the hepatic veins
    c. enlarged caudate lobe
    d. ascites and hepatomegaly

Fill-in-the-Blank

1. The junction of the splenic and superior mesenteric veins forms the _____.

2. The _____ portal vein branches into anterior and posterior segments, and the _____ portal vein branches into medial and lateral segments.

3. Hepatic veins _____ in size as they approach the diaphragm.

4. The patient and transducer position that provides optimal visualization of the splenic vein and artery is the _____.

5. Using a higher frequency transducer during portal venous duplex examination can allow for better imaging of anterior abdominal wall _____ and assessing the liver surface for _____.

6. In patients with portal hypertension, congestive heart failure, constrictive pericarditis, and portal vein thrombosis, portal vein diameters can be expected to _____.

7. Portal vein flow is normally _____ in direction with constant antegrade flow throughout the cardiac cycle.

8. Patients with tricuspid regurgitation, right-sided congestive heart failure, or arteriovenous fistulas may present with _____ flow in the portal vein.

9. Both the _____ and _____ veins demonstrate monophasic flow with slight pulsatility that is directed toward the liver.

10. Hepatic veins exhibit _____ waveforms that correspond to cyclic pressure changes within the heart.

11. With ingestion of food, portal vein flow velocities _____, whereas hepatic artery velocities _____.

12. Patient size, right atrial pressure, and fluid overload or heart failure affect IVC _____.

13. Portal hypertension becomes significant when the pressure gradient between the portal vein and IVC exceeds _____.

14. Until recently, the most common cause of cirrhosis was alcohol abuse; however, _____ infection now accounts for a larger percentage of cases.

15. Cirrhosis would be considered a(n) _____ cause of portal hypertension.

16. Sonographic findings of portal hypertension can include portal vein diameter greater than _____ mm and _____ flow in the portal vein.

17. The most specific finding of portal hypertension is the detection of _____.

18. Color duplex imaging findings of an enlarged hepatic artery with high-velocity, turbulent flow, and a tortuous "corkscrew" appearance is referred to as _____.

19. Penetrating trauma, iatrogenic trauma due to liver biopsy, transhepatic cholangiography, and transhepatic catheterization of the bile ducts or portal veins may create a(n) _____, which may cause life-threatening portal hypertension.

20. An abnormal connection between the portal vein and hepatic vein is termed as _____, which can lead to an increased pulsatility in the portal vein waveform.

21. A TIPS is typically placed to the management of uncontrollable _____ and refractory ascites.

22. If portal vein thrombosis persists without lysis, development of periportal collateral veins increases and is known as _____.

23. A spectrum of hepatic disorders that occurs in the setting of right-sided heart failure and causes an accumulation of deoxygenated blood, parenchymal atrophy, necrosis, collagen deposition, and ultimately fibrosis is termed _____.

24. Malignant tumor infiltration, parasitic mass, or extrinsic compression from a neighboring mass can result in _____ hepatic venous outflow obstruction.

25. A patient with fatigue, abdominal swelling, and signs and symptoms of portal hypertension but with patency of the large hepatic and portal veins would likely be diagnosed with _____.

Short Answer

1. List the indications for hepatoportal duplex ultrasound.

2. What are the key differences between portal veins and hepatic veins within the liver?

3. What anatomic features of the liver should be documented during hepatoportal duplex examination?

4. What are the major limitations affecting the success of the hepatoportal duplex examination?

5. What are the normal findings in a well-functioning TIPS?

IMAGE EVALUATION/PATHOLOGY

Review the images and answer the following questions.

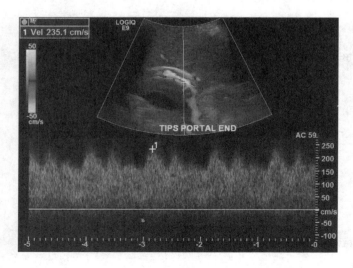

1. This Doppler waveform was taken from the mid-region of a TIPS. What do these findings suggest?

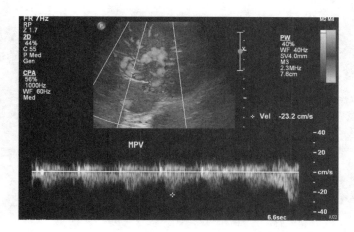

2. This image demonstrates color Doppler imaging of the main portal vein area. What do these findings suggest?

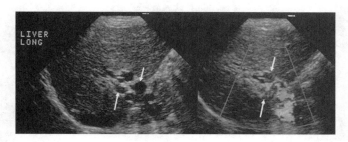

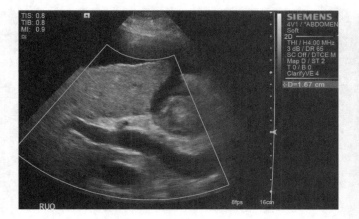

3. This image shows another view of the porta hepatis with color-flow Doppler. Describe the findings.

CASE STUDY

Review the information and answer the following questions.

1. A 58-year-old male presents to the vascular lab for hepatoportal duplex examination with a history of alcoholism. These images were obtained during his examination. Describe the findings. What pathology do these images suggest?

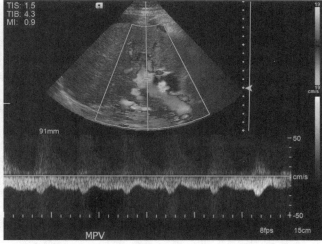

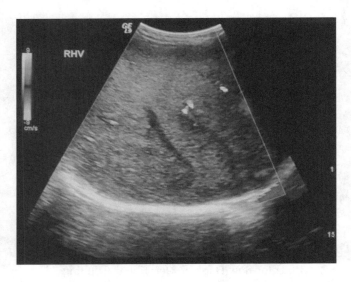

2. A 23-year-old female presents to the vascular lab
   for hepatoportal duplex examination. The patient
   presents with right upper quadrant pain, jaundice,
   ascites, and hepatomegaly and has a history of oral
   contraceptive use. The above image was obtained
   during her examination. Describe the findings in this
   image. What is suggested by her clinical presentation
   and imaging findings?

Evaluation of Kidney and Liver Transplants

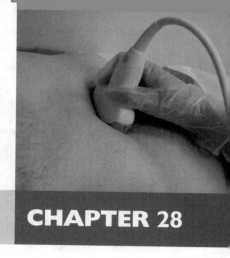

REVIEW OF GLOSSARY TERMS

Matching

Match the key terms with their definitions.

KEY TERMS

1. _____ allograft

2. _____ orthotopic transplant

3. _____ transplant rejection

4. _____ immunosuppression drugs

5. _____ arteriovenous fistula

6. _____ pseudoaneurysm

DEFINITION

a. The failure of a transplant occurring secondary to the formation of antidonor antibodies by the recipient. It can lead to loss of the transplant

b. A connection between an artery and a vein, usually posttraumatic in origin

c. Drugs used to inhibit the body's formation of antibodies to the allograft

d. Develops secondary to a tear in the arterial wall allowing extravasation of blood from the arterial lumen, which is contained by a compacted rim of surrounding soft tissue

e. A transplant that is placed in the same anatomic location as the native organ

f. Any tissue transplanted from one human to another human

CHAPTER REVIEW

Multiple Choice

Complete each question by circling the best answer.

1. Which of the following is NOT a symptom of kidney graft failure?
   a. elevated red blood count
   b. fever and chills
   c. elevated serum creatinine level
   d. pain and tenderness

2. Where are kidney transplants most frequently placed?
   a. normal kidney position
   b. right iliac fossa position
   c. left iliac fossa position
   d. right posterior position

3. In a DD kidney transplant, which vessel anastomosis is performed?
   a. donor aortic wall and recipient external iliac artery
   b. donor aortic wall and recipient internal iliac artery
   c. recipient renal artery and donor external iliac artery
   d. recipient external iliac artery and donor main renal artery

4. Which of the following is a renal transplant complication that is relatively common in the postsurgical period?
   a. superinfection
   b. urinoma
   c. lymphocele
   d. ureteral occlusion

5. What is the optimal time frame to perform a baseline sonogram in renal transplant patient?
   a. 6 hours
   b. 12 hours
   c. 24 hours
   d. 48 hours

6. How long after transplantation does the kidney reach maximal size?
   a. 12 months
   b. 6 months
   c. 4 months
   d. 2 months

7. Which sonographic image would best demonstrate the presence of a urinoma?
   a. transverse superior to the kidney
   b. sagittal at mid-kidney
   c. transverse bladder
   d. oblique view of lower pole of kidney and bladder

8. What is normal arterial RI in a transplanted kidney?
   a. 0.5
   b. 0.7
   c. 0.9
   d. 1.0

9. Which velocity is critical to accurately calculate the RI?
   a. early diastolic
   b. mid-diastolic
   c. end diastolic
   d. systolic

10. What pattern of color display in the interlobar arteries is consistent with normal flow?
    a. flow with minimal diminishment at end diastole
    b. lack of flow at end diastole
    c. flashy and pulsatile
    d. minimal flow at end diastole

11. When does graft loss caused by rejection occur?
    a. 3 months
    b. 6 months
    c. 9 months
    d. 12 months

12. What is the medical term for sudden cessation of urine production?
    a. anuria
    b. oliguria
    c. polyuria
    d. hematuria

13. Which of the following is NOT a risk factor for development of ATN?
    a. ischemic time
    b. hypertension
    c. donor illness
    d. nonheart beating surgery

14. Which of the following best describes a perinephric fluid collection with multiple thin septations?
    a. hematoma
    b. urinoma
    c. hydronephrosis
    d. lymphocele

15. Which of the following best describes sonographic duplex findings consistent with renal artery thrombosis (RAT)?
    a. anechoic lumen with low-resistance flow pattern
    b. anechoic lumen with high-resistance flow pattern
    c. intraluminal echoes with low-resistance flow pattern
    d. intraluminal echoes with absence of flow

16. With which of the following transplant complications does enlargement of the kidney with decreased renal cortical echogenicity most consistent?
    a. renal artery thrombosis
    b. renal vein thrombosis
    c. renal artery stenosis
    d. lymphocele

17. What is the most common vascular complication following renal transplantation?
    a. renal artery thrombus
    b. renal vein thrombus
    c. renal artery stenosis
    d. renal artery kink

18. What do Doppler criteria consistent with RAS of >50% to 60% in transplanted kidney include?
    a. PSV >250 cm/s
    b. PSV ratio ≤2.0 to 3.0
    c. AT <70 to 80 ms
    d. lack of end-diastolic flow

19. Which of the following is NOT a Doppler characteristic of an AVF?
    a. area of color aliasing
    b. soft tissue color bruit
    c. high velocity in both systole and diastole
    d. low velocity in both systole and diastole

20. Which type of anastomosis is performed for the arterial anastomosis of hepatic artery in liver transplants?
    a. end to end
    b. side to side
    c. fish mouth
    d. piggy back

21. Which of the following is the most common cause of liver transplant loss?
    a. rejection
    b. biliary complication
    c. surgical technique
    d. vascular cause

22. Which of the following is NOT a contraindication for liver transplantation?
    a. renal malignancy
    b. untreated infection
    c. hemochromatosis
    d. CHF and COPD

23. What is the preferred anastomosis of donor CBD?
    a. common hepatic duct
    b. common bile duct
    c. duodenum
    d. jejunum

24. What is the best patient "window" for sonographic duplex assessment of hepatic transplant?
    a. infracostal
    b. midline
    c. subcostal
    d. intercostal

25. What is the most common vascular complication of liver transplantation?
    a. hepatic artery thrombosis
    b. hepatic artery stenosis
    c. hepatic artery pseudoaneurysm
    d. portal vein thrombosis

26. A liver transplant patient presents to the vascular lab for evaluation after core needle biopsy. Which of the following would be a concern in this patient?
    a. hepatic artery thrombosis
    b. intrahepatic artery pseudoaneurysm
    c. portal vein thrombosis
    d. hepatic artery stenosis

27. Upon duplex evaluation of a recent liver transplant, tardus parvus waveforms are noted in the interparenchymal hepatic arteries. Which of the following would be a concern in this patient?
    a. hepatic artery thrombosis
    b. intrahepatic artery pseudoaneurysm
    c. portal vein thrombosis
    d. hepatic artery stenosis

28. What would be suspected in a liver transplant patient with signs of early liver failure and portal hypertension?
    a. hepatic artery thrombosis
    b. intrahepatic artery pseudoaneurysm
    c. portal vein thrombosis
    d. hepatic artery stenosis

29. A liver transplant patient presents to the vascular lab with worsening liver function. Upon duplex evaluation, velocities in the main portal vein reach 200 cm/s. What do these findings suggest?
    a. portal vein stenosis
    b. hepatic artery thrombosis
    c. portal vein thrombosis
    d. portal vein pseudoaneurysm

30. A liver transplant patient presents to the vascular lab for follow up. Upon questioning, the patient indicates he has been experiencing lower extremity swelling. Which of the following would be of concern to the vascular technologist?
    a. portal vein thrombosis
    b. hepatic artery thrombosis
    c. inferior vena cava thrombosis
    d. hepatic vein thrombosis

Fill-in-the-Blank

1. Organs for transplantations are from either a _____ donor (DD) or a _____ donor (LRD).

2. Diabetes mellitus, autosomal dominant polycystic kidney disease, glomerulonephritis, hypertension, atherosclerosis, and systemic lupus erythematous can all lead to _____.

3. Anuria, rising creatinine level, pain, tenderness, and fever are all symptoms related to _____.

4. The oval piece of donor's aortic wall that contains the main renal artery is called a _____.

5. The donor renal artery is directly anastomosed to the recipient's _____ with an end-to-side approach, whereas the donor renal vein is anastomosed to the recipient's _____ in an end-to-side approach.

6. Because of relaxation in donor criteria, _____ often presents earlier and is more severe than previously.

7. Kidney graft failure caused by acute tubular necrosis, pyelonephritis, rejection, and drug toxicity are best managed _____.

8. Mild _____ is a normal finding postrenal transplantation.

9. Hypercoagulable states, hypotension, intraoperative trauma, mismatch of vessel size, and vascular kinking are risk factors for _____.

10. The presenting symptom of a patient with renal artery stenosis after a renal transplant is severe _____.

11. Extrahepatic malignancy, untreated infection, metastatic hepatocellular carcinoma, active substance abuse, cholangiocarcinoma, and advanced age are some of the _____ for liver transplantation.

12. Liver transplantation is the only available option for patients with acute or chronic _____ who are unresponsive to medical therapy.

13. Criteria used to rank patients for liver transplant are _____ and _____ score.

14. If a patient has a choledochojejunostomy, bile will drain directly into the _____.

15. Owing to a shortage of donor livers, partial liver transplants from living donors are more frequently performed with the _____ lobe of the liver used a transplant.

16. In liver transplantation, hepatic artery stenosis or occlusion is often associated with _____ pathology owing to sole blood supply.

17. The hepatic artery anastomosis is created with a "_____" technique whereby the smaller vessel's walls are split and sewn over the larger vessel.

18. A patient presents with poor liver function tests and biliary ischemia; these symptoms would be consistent with _____.

19. The Doppler waveform in a hepatic artery pseudoaneurysm is _____, showing a typical mix of arterial and venous signals.

20. When evaluating for possible portal vein thrombosis, the sonographer should use _____ because of the low velocity or absence of flow.

Short Answer

1. Describe why cadaveric donor allografts continue to increase in graft survival.

2. List at least five causes of true hydronephrosis in a transplanted kidney.

3. What are the common nonvascular postoperative complications after liver transplantation.

IMAGE EVALUATION/PATHOLOGY

Review the images and answer the following questions.

1. These images were taken from the patient shortly after renal transplant. What is demonstrated in these images?

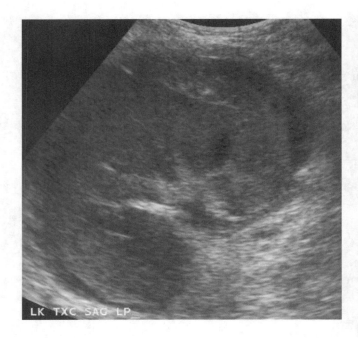

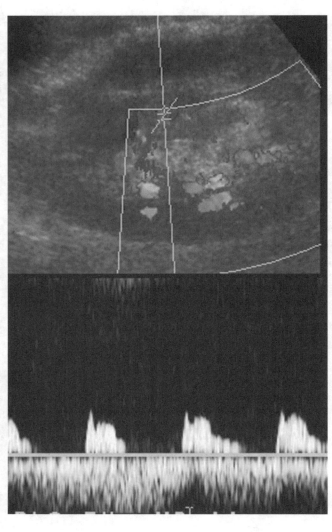

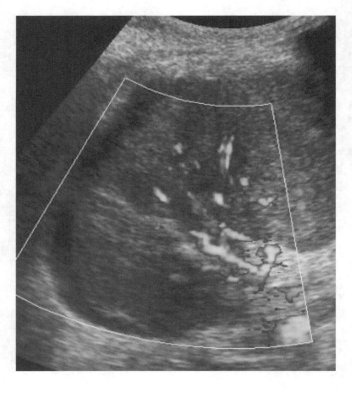

2. These images were taken from the same patient several days postoperatively after renal transplant. The patient presents with severe uncontrolled hypertension. What are these images consistent with?

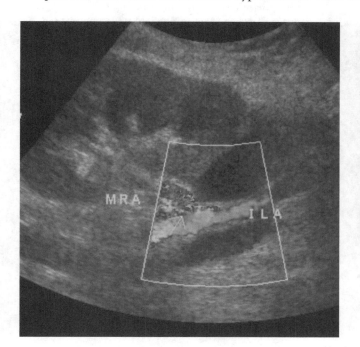

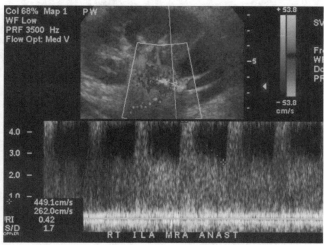

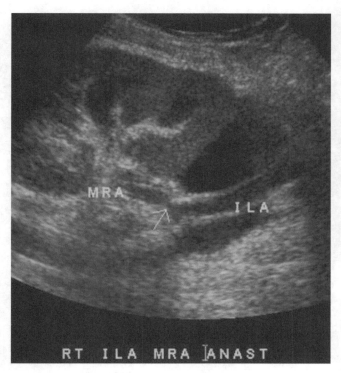

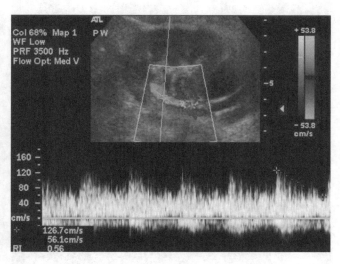

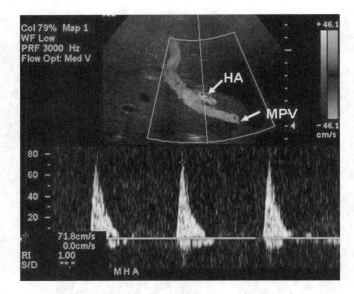

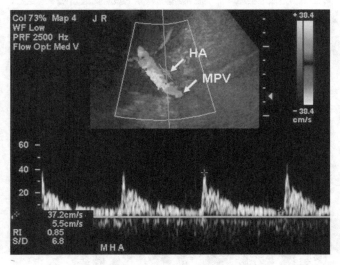

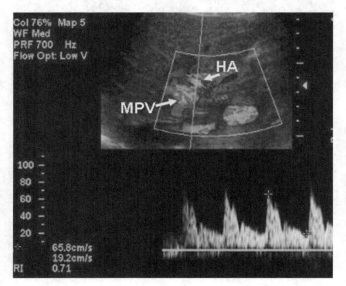

3. This series of images was taken in the main hepatic artery after liver transplant. The first image is immediately postoperative, the next image is 2 days postoperative, and the last image is 4 days postoperative. What do these images demonstrate?

CASE STUDY

Review the information and answer the following questions.

1. A 35-year-old female patient who is approximately 3 months post-DD renal transplant presents to the emergency department with oliguria. The lab tests confirm increase in serum creatinine and blood urea nitrogen. She is sent to the ultrasound department for evaluation. As a sonographer, what would you expect to find sonographically, and what is the most likely cause for these symptoms?

2. A 57-year-old male patient with a past history of early-stage hepatocellular carcinoma treated with a single lobe LRD 3 weeks ago presents for follow-up complaining of nausea and vomiting with increasing jaundice. After drawing LFTs, the patient is sent to the ultrasound lab for evaluation. What types of vascular and nonvascular complications could cause the patient's symptoms?

PART SEVEN

MISCELLANEOUS

Intraoperative Duplex Ultrasound

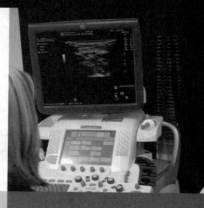

CHAPTER 29

REVIEW OF GLOSSARY TERMS

Matching

Match the key terms with their definitions.

KEY TERMS

1. _____ autologous/autogenous

2. _____ endarterectomy

3. _____ infrainguinal

4. _____ prosthetic

5. _____ revascularization

6. _____ sterile technique

7. _____ surveillance

8. _____ visceral

DEFINITION

a. Below the inguinal level; procedure performed below the groin
b. Restoration of blood flow to an organ or area by way of bypass, endarterectomy, or angioplasty and stenting
c. Keeping a watch over; periodically monitoring patency and functioning by some means
d. Removal of plaque, intima, and part of media of an artery to restore normal flow through the diseased segment
e. Means by which a surgical field is isolated from nonsterile or contaminated materials
f. Pertaining to the viscera (intestines or kidneys)
g. Self-produced or from the same organisms
h. A device replacing an absent or a damaged part; a man-made tube used for the bypass procedure

CHAPTER REVIEW

Multiple Choice

Complete each question by circling the best answer.

1. Which of the following is considered the "gold standard" for intraoperative assessment of any type of revascularization?
   a. duplex ultrasound
   b. arteriography
   c. CW Doppler only
   d. palpation

2. Which duplex ultrasound system requirements would be best suited for intraoperative assessment?
   a. portable systems with high-frequency transducers
   b. high-end systems with large-array transducers
   c. grayscale-only systems with high-frequency transducers
   d. large systems with a variety of transducers

3. What is the primary role of the vascular technologist during intraoperative procedures?
   a. Manipulation of the transducer in the sterile field as well as system operation
   b. Manipulation of the transducer in the sterile field only
   c. Operation of the ultrasound system as the vascular surgeon manipulates the transducer
   d. The vascular technologist does not participate during intraoperative procedures.

4. In general, when performing an intraoperative assessment, which of the following imaging techniques is best?
   a. grayscale imaging only
   b. spectral Doppler analysis only
   c. combination of grayscale, color, and spectral Doppler
   d. color Doppler assessment only

5. What is NOT a benefit of angiography in the intraoperative assessment of carotid endarterectomy?
   a. Ability to visualize the intracranial carotid artery
   b. Ability to visualize the extracranial internal carotid artery
   c. The use of contrast is not needed.
   d. It offers physiologic data as well as anatomic data.

6. During intraoperative assessment of carotid endarterectomy, spectral Doppler demonstrated velocities of 200 cm/s in the internal carotid artery, whereas velocities in the common carotid artery were 70 cm/s. Based on these findings, which of the following is likely to occur?
   a. closure of the surgical site with no further investigation
   b. closure of the surgical site with duplex assessment performed 1 day postoperatively
   c. repeat intraoperative duplex assessment 30 minutes later
   d. revision of the surgical site with repeat duplex assessment after revision

7. Which of the following duplex ultrasound findings is NOT associated with platelet aggregation?
   a. hypoechoic or anechoic material adjacent to vessel wall
   b. focal elevation in peak systolic velocities
   c. increased velocity ratios
   d. linear object visualized parallel to vessel walls

8. Upon duplex assessment of a carotid endarterectomy site, shadowing is noted in the proximal internal carotid artery. What is the most likely cause of this shadowing?
   a. residual atherosclerotic plaquing at the carotid bulb
   b. artifact from the prosthetic patch at the endarterectomy site
   c. occlusion of the internal carotid artery from neointimal hyperplasia
   d. gain setting too low on the ultrasound system

9. Which of the following can lead to complications or failure of an infrainguinal bypass graft?
   a. inadequate arterial inflow
   b. use of prosthetic material below the knee
   c. significant disease in the outflow vessels
   d. all the above

10. Which of the following is a main advantage of intraoperative duplex assessment of infrainguinal bypass grafts?

    a. Complete anatomic evaluation of the graft.

    b. Identification of retained valves.

    c. Physiologic information is gathered as well as anatomic.

    d. Shadowing caused by prosthetic material will enhance the image.

11. What is the preferred bypass conduit for infrainguinal revascularization?

    a. Dacron material

    b. PTFE material

    c. autologous material

    d. All materials are equally preferred.

12. What may abnormally low graft velocities in an infrainguinal bypass graft indicate?

    a. poor inflow vessels

    b. poor outflow vessels

    c. proximal anastomosis attachment failure

    d. arteriovenous fistulae

13. Which criterion is used most often when assessing whether to revise an infrainguinal bypass graft during intraoperative assessment?

    a. PSV >180 cm/s and velocity ratio >2.5

    b. PWV <150 cm/s and velocity ratio <1.0

    c. PSV >125 cm/s and velocity ratio >4.0

    d. PSV >250 cm/s and velocity ratio >2.5

14. During intraoperative duplex assessment of a lower extremity bypass graft, turbulent flow is noted in the mid-thigh with elevated diastolic flow noted in the proximal thigh. What are these findings consistent with?

    a. dissection

    b. shelf lesion

    c. intimal flap

    d. arteriovenous fistula

15. Why may intraoperative duplex ultrasound evaluation of renal artery bypass be preferred over angiography?

    a. Failure of renal artery bypass frequently results in death.

    b. Duplex ultrasound avoids the use of contrast in a renal compromised patient.

    c. It has been shown to be more accurate than angiography.

    d. It does not require the presence of a technologist to operate the equipment.

16. Why is intraoperative duplex ultrasound NOT used in aortoiliac reconstructions?

    a. Small defects are not as patency threatening in these large vessels.

    b. Because of surgical technique, defects aren't detectable on ultrasound.

    c. Large amounts of bowel gas make imaging impossible.

    d. Ultrasound devices aren't configured for use in the abdomen.

17. What velocity is typically used as an indication to revise a renal artery bypass during intraoperative assessment?

    a. >180 cm/s

    b. >275 cm/s

    c. >200 cm/s

    d. <100 cm/s

18. During a superior mesenteric artery bypass intraoperative evaluation, an intimal flap is discovered and velocities were 300 cm/s. What would likely occur with this graft?

    a. Normal graft findings

    b. Graft revision would be indicated.

    c. Graft failure is imminent even with intervention.

    d. Graft will require increased monitoring.

19. What is a common venous procedure in which intraoperative monitoring is routinely used?

    a. DVT anticoagulation treatment

    b. superficial thrombophlebitis ablation

    c. varicose vein stripping and ligation

    d. endovenous laser therapy (EVLT)

20. What is an evolving ultrasound technology used for guidance of endovenous interventions?

    a. IVUS

    b. EVLT

    c. AVF

    d. PTFE

Fill-in-the-Blank

1. A typical transducer used during an intraoperative procedure would be a _____ frequency, linear array.

2. During an intraoperative procedure, a sterile _____ is placed over the transducer once filled with sterile gel, and bubbles are removed to reduce interference.

3. In duplex assessment of infrainguinal revascularization, injection of papaverine into the bypass is helpful in minimizing the effects of _____.

4. Because prosthetic materials absorb _____, intraoperative scanning of these materials is virtually impossible; however, prosthetic _____ in carotid endarterectomy can usually be worked around.

5. For the vascular technologist to assist in the operating room, they must have familiarity with _____ technique.

6. Carotid endarterectomy is one of the most common operations performed by vascular surgeons and typically has stroke rates below _____%; however, there remains some value of intraoperative assessment to minimize residual _____.

7. Continuous-wave Doppler is probably the most commonly used assessment during carotid endarterectomy; however, _____-wave Doppler or _____ imaging are being shown to be effective for intraoperative assessment.

8. During duplex assessment of carotid endarterectomy, velocities are obtained from all the carotid arteries, and B-mode images are closely examined for wall _____.

9. Plaque remaining in the proximal internal carotid artery or distal common carotid artery after endarterectomy, which appears as an abrupt edge or outcropping, is often referred to as a(n)_____.

10. A(n) _____ is another complication of endarterectomy and is often revised if in excess of _____ mm.

11. Infrainguinal revascularization can be perfumed for claudication or _____.

12. While carotid endarterectomy is fairly standardized, issues are common with infrainguinal revascularization because there are many _____ in the performance of the procedure.

13. The so-called "_____" veins are more prone to abnormalities that can result in failure of an infrainguinal bypass graft.

14. To identify retained valves, scarred areas, arteriovenous fistula, or platelet aggregation, duplex scanning during lower extremity bypass allows the _____ of the bypass to be evaluated.

15. Findings that prompt revision of lower extremity bypass grafts include a peak systolic velocity greater than _____ cm/s and a velocity ratio greater than _____.

16. On duplex assessment of an infrainguinal bypass, an increased velocity shift was noted; however, the lumen of the conduit appears anechoic—this could be the result of _____.

17. Duplex sonography has distinct advantages over angiography in the assessment of visceral revascularizations, including the ability to visualize small vessels and the lack of the need for _____, particularly for patients with poor renal function.

18. In renal bypass assessment, velocities of _____ cm/s by duplex scanning were an indication for revision.

19. Abnormal intraoperative duplex studies of mesenteric bypass grafts have been associated with early _____, graft _____, and even death.

20. Criteria for normal results of a mesenteric bypass graft include peak systolic velocities below _____ cm/s for the celiac artery and _____ cm/s for the superior mesenteric artery, a velocity ratio less than _____ and no technical defects.

Short Answer

1. Describe the preparation that is necessary for both the surgical site and the ultrasound system when used in the operating room. What is the role of the vascular technologist?

2. Compare the advantages and drawbacks of angiography versus duplex scanning in the intraoperative environment.

IMAGE EVALUATION/PATHOLOGY

Review the images and answer the following questions.

1. You are assisting a vascular surgeon during carotid endarterectomy. During the procedure, these images were obtained.
   a. Describe the findings in these images.
   b. Based on these findings, what would the next course of action likely be?

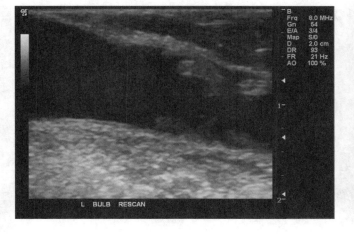
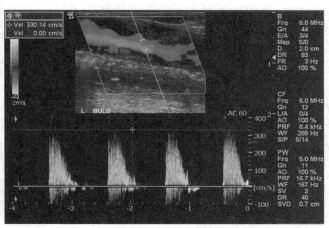

CASE STUDY

Review the information and answer the following questions.

1. A 65-year-old male is undergoing infrainguinal bypass grafting on the left leg. The vascular surgeon is using autologous veins for the bypass. What specific complications should you be concerned about during the intraoperative evaluation? What findings would likely warrant reexamination and/or revision of the graft?

2. During intraoperative duplex assessment of a superior mesenteric bypass graft, velocities near the distal anastomosis were observed to reach 350 cm/s. What are these findings consistent with? What might the consequences of these findings be?

Hemodialysis Access Grafts and Fistulae

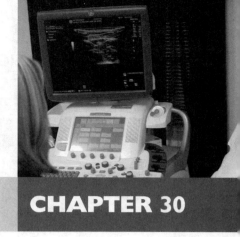

CHAPTER 30

REVIEW OF GLOSSARY TERMS

Matching

Match the key terms with their definitions.

KEY TERMS

1. _____ hemodialysis access

2. _____ arteriovenous fistula

3. _____ arteriovenous graft

DEFINITION

a. Any connection between an artery and a vein; may be congenital, traumatic, or acquired

b. A type of hemodialysis access that uses a prosthetic conduit to connect an artery to a vein to allow for dialysis

c. Also known as vascular access, a surgically created connection between an artery and a vein to allow for removal of toxic products from the blood by dialysis

ANATOMY AND PHYSIOLOGY REVIEW

Image Labeling

Complete the labels in the images that follow.

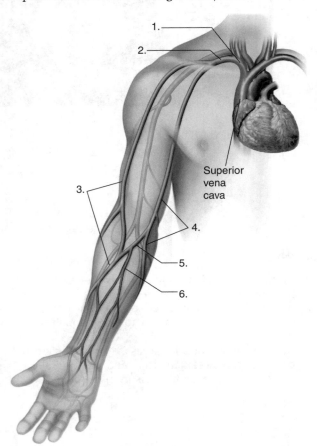

1. Veins in the upper extremity.

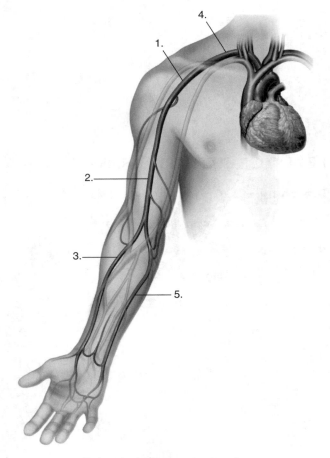

2. Arteries in the upper extremity.

CHAPTER REVIEW

Multiple Choice

Complete each question by circling the best answer.

1. The goal of the Kidney Dialysis Outcomes Quality Initiative and the Fistula First Breakthrough Initiative was to increase and expand the creation of which of the following?
   a. prosthetic hemodialysis access grafts
   b. autogenous hemodialysis access fistulae
   c. lower extremity hemodialysis access
   d. central venous port access

2. What is the most common cause of maturation failure of dialysis access fistulae?
   a. small or suboptimal veins
   b. venous outflow stenosis
   c. arterial inflow stenosis
   d. arterial steal syndrome

3. Which of the following should be included during the physical examination for preoperative artery mapping for dialysis fistula creation?
   a. bilateral arm blood pressure measurements
   b. pulse exam of brachial, radial, and ulnar arteries
   c. Allen test for palmar arch assessment
   d. all the above

4. Which of the following is NOT a finding suggestive of a central venous stenosis or occlusion?
   a. arm edema
   b. prominent chest wall veins
   c. painful, cool, pale hand
   d. presence of arm collaterals

5. Which of the following describes the proper patient positioning for upper extremity venous evaluation prior to fistula creation?
   a. supine with arm elevated
   b. supine or sitting with arm dependent
   c. standing with weight held in arm to be examined
   d. Trendelenburg with feet elevated

6. With what does standard protocol for evaluation of the upper extremity arteries and veins for fistula creation begin?
   a. veins of dominant arm
   b. veins of nondominant arm
   c. arteries of dominant arm
   d. arteries of nondominant arm

7. What is the acceptable size for upper extremity arteries before fistula creation?
   a. >2.0 mm
   b. >2.5 mm
   c. <3.0 mm
   d. <2.0 mm

8. All Doppler studies should be performed at an angle of _____ or less, even if actual velocities are not recorded to achieve adequate Doppler signals.
   a. 75 degrees
   b. 60 degrees
   c. 90 degrees
   d. 0 degree

9. What is the acceptable minimum vein diameter for favorable fistula creation?
   a. 2.0 mm
   b. 1.5 mm
   c. 2.5 mm
   d. 1.0 mm

10. Which of the following should venous Doppler signals from central veins NOT display?
    a. respiratory phasicity
    b. cardiac pulsatility
    c. augmentation
    d. continuous flow

11. What is a type of fistula created by connecting the posterior branch of the radial artery to the cephalic vein?
    a. Brescia–Cimino fistula
    b. transposition fistula
    c. snuffbox fistula
    d. Berman–Gentile fistula

12. The most common upper arm access is made between the cephalic vein and which artery?
    a. subclavian artery
    b. brachial artery
    c. axillary artery
    d. brachiocephalic artery

13. Approximately how long should it take an autogenous fistula to mature?
    a. 8 to 12 weeks
    b. 1 to 3 days
    c. 6 to 8 months
    d. 1 to 2 years

14. During evaluation of the upper extremity either before or after fistula creation, the examination room should be kept warm to avoid what?
    a. vasodilation
    b. vasospasm
    c. the use of coupling gel
    d. ultrasound equipment failure

15. Which of the following is NOT included in a physical examination of a patient with a current AV fistula?
    a. assessment of thrill
    b. assessment for edema or redness
    c. bilateral radial blood pressures
    d. visual inspection for focal dilations and collateral veins

16. During duplex assessment of the hemodialysis fistula, what should Doppler settings be adjusted to detect?
    a. low flow
    b. continuous flow
    c. intermittent flow
    d. high flow

17. Which of the following describes how volumetric flow is calculated?
    a. time average velocity/PSV
    b. time average velocity × area × 60
    c. time average velocity × vessel diameter
    d. PSV − EDV / PSV

18. What can remaining valve leaflets that project into the lumen of a fistula become a source for?
    a. dissection
    b. pseudoaneurysm development
    c. stenosis development
    d. calcium deposition

19. A patient presents to the vascular lab for follow-up evaluation of a dialysis fistula. Velocities within the fistula are 40 cm/s. What are these findings consistent with?
    a. normal fistula function
    b. fistula pseudoaneurysm
    c. perigraft mass
    d. inflow artery stenosis

20. What should be the approximate normal volume flow in a fistula?
    a. 200 mL/min
    b. 500 mL/min
    c. 800 mL/min
    d. 100 mL/min

Fill-in-the-Blank

1. The goal of arteriovenous access is to provide long-term hemodialysis access with a _____ frequency of reintervention and a low _____ rate.

2. _____ access has been the preferred first-line therapy because it has superior patency rates and lower complication rates compared to _____.

3. AV fistulas have higher long-term patency rates; however, they suffer from lower _____ rates and higher early _____ rates.

4. Placement of central venous catheters, pacemakers, defibrillators, or prior mastectomy with lymph node dissection may _____ the creation of an arteriovenous hemodialysis fistula.

5. AV fistula creation is usually first attempted in the _____ upper extremity as far _____ as possible.

6. Atherosclerosis is uncommon in the upper extremities, but when it occurs, it most commonly affects the _____ artery.

7. To maximally dilate the veins, a(n) _____ may be used either just below the antecubital fossa for forearm veins or at the axillary level for upper arm veins.

8. Patency of veins should be confirmed both with transducer _____ and with spectral Doppler waveforms.

9. A dilated, easily palpable, usable fistula with a flow rate of >350 cc/min defines a fistula that has _____.

10. A partially or noncompressible vein suggests the presence of an occluding _____ within the vein lumen, making it _____ as an autogenous conduit.

11. A Brescia–Cimino fistula is the most frequently created fistula and involves the _____ vein and the _____ artery at the wrist.

12. Because of its deep location, the _____ vein requires that it be transposed and juxtaposed to a distal artery to create an AV fistula.

13. While performing duplex assessment either preoperatively or after hemodialysis fistula placement, the examination room should be kept warm to avoid _____.

14. To assess for edema, redness, presence of collateral veins, rotation of access sites, and focal dilations, the arm should be _____ by the technologist before duplex assessment.

15. Presence of perigraft masses, pseudoaneurysms, stenotic valves, and intimal flaps should be assessed during _____ imaging evaluation of a dialysis fistula.

16. When stenosis is found, spectral Doppler velocities should be measured _____, _____, and _____ the area of interest.

17. When measuring volume flow rates of a hemodialysis fistula, the _____ is used and is best measured over _____ cardiac cycles to obtain an accurate calculation.

18. As fistulas mature, they typically become tortuous and can become aneurysmal, thus requiring larger amounts of _____ to maintain proper skin contact over these surface irregularities.

19. If a hemodialysis fistula has a volume flow measurement <500 mL/min, this would indicate _____ in the fistula.

20. _____ and _____ stenoses account for the majority of access complications.

Short Answer

1. Why is it important for the inflow artery to a dialysis access fistula to be free of calcifications and/or atherosclerosis?

2. When would it be appropriate to use the lower extremity for fistula creation? What vessels can be used?

3. List the indications for fistula assessment after it has been placed.

4. Describe the symptoms and sonographic findings associated with arterial steal syndrome.

5. Describe the sonographic findings in a normal hemodialysis fistula, including arterial inflow within the fistula and outflow vein.

IMAGE EVALUATION/PATHOLOGY

Review the images and answer the following questions.

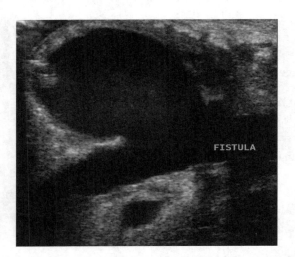

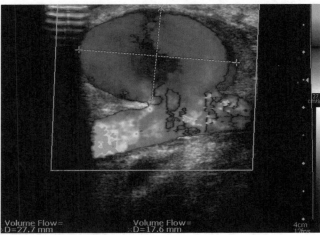

1. The images shown on the left were taken from the mid-forearm. What do these images demonstrate?

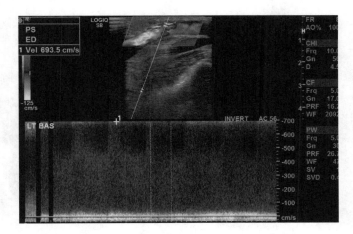

2. This image demonstrates the anastomosis of a dialysis access fistula. What do this image demonstrate?

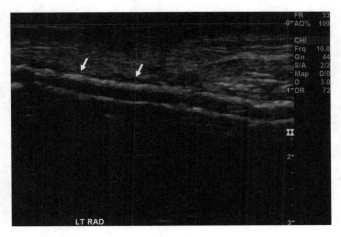

3. This image was obtained from the forearm of a diabetic patient. What do this image demonstrate?

CASE STUDY

Review the information and answer the following questions.

1. A right-handed patient presents to the vascular laboratory for upper extremity evaluation prior to hemodialysis access creation. What protocol would you use to evaluate this patient, and what criteria would you use to determine whether the vessels are adequate for fistula placement?

2. A patient presents to the vascular lab with elevated venous pressure during dialysis. What findings would you expect on your duplex assessment of this fistula?

Evaluation of Penile Blood Flow

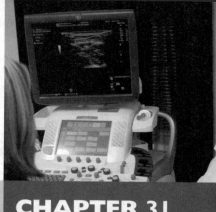

CHAPTER 31

REVIEW OF GLOSSARY TERMS

Matching

Match the key terms with their definitions.

KEY TERMS

1. _____ cavernosal artery

2. _____ corpora cavernosa

3. _____ erectile dysfunction

4. _____ penile brachial index

5. _____ Peyronie's disease

6. _____ priapism

7. _____ tunica albuginea

DEFINITION

a. The persistent ability to achieve or maintain an erection suitable for sexual intercourse; also known as impotence

b. Full or partial erection that continues more than 4 hours beyond sexual stimulation and orgasm or is unrelated to sexual stimulation

c. One of three terminal branches of the common penile artery. It supplies blood flow to the corpora cavernosa

d. An acquired penile deformity caused by fibrosis of the tunica albuginea, resulting in plaque formation

e. Two paired areas of spongy erectile tissue

f. The tough fibrous layer of connective tissue that surrounds the corpora cavernosa of the penis

g. The ratio of penile systolic pressure and brachial systolic pressure

ANATOMY AND PHYSIOLOGY REVIEW

Image Labeling

Complete the labels in the images that follow.

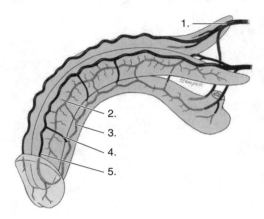

1. The arterial vasculature of the penis.

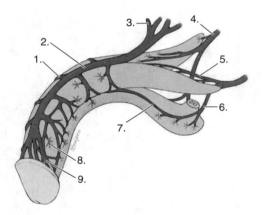

2. The venous vasculature of the penis.

CHAPTER REVIEW

Multiple Choice

Complete each question by circling the best answer.

1. Where does the arterial vascular supply to the penis originate?
   a. common iliac artery
   b. internal iliac artery
   c. external iliac artery
   d. common femoral artery

2. What are the two masses of erectile tissue composed of multiple sinusoidal chambers?
   a. tunica albuginea
   b. corpora spongiosa
   c. corpora cavernosa
   d. bulbourethral sinusoids

3. Which vessel supplies the glans and other nonerectile tissue?
   a. cavernous artery
   b. bulbourethral artery
   c. corporal artery
   d. dorsal artery

4. What is a connection of veins that drains the dorsal veins of the penis into the internal iliac or internal pudendal vein?
   a. periprostatic plexus
   b. corpus spongiosum
   c. periurethral plexus
   d. cavernous sinus

5. What results from the plaque formations associated with Peyronie's disease?
   a. penile curvature
   b. priapism
   c. arterial stenosis
   d. penile straightening

6. What is recommended all patient with Peyronie's disease have prior to performing invasive treatments?
   a. duplex Doppler ultrasound only
   b. duplex Doppler ultrasound with intracavernosal injection
   c. CT scan with intracavernosal injection
   d. intraurethral ultrasound

7. What percent of erectile dysfunction is attributed to vascular disease?
   a. 5%
   b. 30%
   c. 50%
   d. 80%

8. Which of the following would increase the risk of arterial causes of erectile dysfunction?
   a. diabetes
   b. hypertension
   c. smoking history
   d. all the above

9. What causes a nonischemic or high-flow priapism?
   a. side effect of erectile dysfunction medication
   b. impaired drainage of blood from the penile bodies
   c. abnormal communication between penile arterial system and cavernosal sinusoids
   d. compartment syndrome within the penis

10. What is the typically cuff width used for a penile pressure?
    a. 10 cm
    b. 12 cm
    c. 2.5 cm
    d. 1 cm

11. How do normal penile systolic pressures compare to brachial systolic pressures?
    a. Penile pressures are higher than brachial pressures.
    b. Penile pressures are less than brachial pressures.
    c. Penile pressures are the same as brachial pressures.
    d. Systolic pressure cannot be measured in a penis.

12. Which of the following is considered normal for a penile–brachial index?
    a. 1.0
    b. >0.7
    c. <0.6
    d. 1.4

13. Which vessels are identified near the central and medial aspects of the corpora cavernosa?
    a. cavernosal arteries
    b. dorsal arteries
    c. bulbourethral arteries
    d. external pudendal arteries

14. What is the purpose of the intracavernosal injection?
    a. To maintain penis in flaccid state.
    b. To decrease arterial inflow to the penis.
    c. To induce and maintain an erection.
    d. To induce contrast agents into penile blood flow.

15. All the following are measured both pre- and postinjection EXCEPT
    a. diameter of cavernosal arteries.
    b. peak systolic velocity of cavernosal arteries.
    c. end-diastolic velocity of cavernosal arteries.
    d. penile length.

16. During grayscale imaging of the corpora cavernosa, a thickened, hyperechoic area is noted on the tunica albuginea. Shadowing is noted as well. What does this likely represent?
    a. fibrous plaque with calcification
    b. calcified arterial wall
    c. normal cavernosal findings
    d. urethral thickening

17. During an erection, to what diameter does the cavernosal artery dilate?
    a. 0.3 mm
    b. 0.7 mm
    c. 1.0 mm
    d. 1.5 mm

18. What occurs in the cavernosal artery following injection?
    a. decrease in PSV and EDV
    b. increase in PSV with little to no diastolic flow
    c. increase in PSV and EDV
    d. decrease in PSV and increase EDV

19. Which of the following velocities is associated with arterial insufficiency postinjection?
    a. <25 cm/s
    b. >13 cm/s
    c. >35 cm/s
    d. >100 cm/s

20. What is a normal value in the deep dorsal vein postinjection?
    a. >4 cm/s
    b. 10 to 20 cm/s
    c. >20 cm/s
    d. <3 cm/s

Fill-in-the-Blank

1. The cavernous, bulbourethral, and dorsal arteries are the terminal branches of the _____ artery.

2. The urethra is contained within the _____.

3. Venous drainage of the penis begins through venules below the tunica albuginea, then through _____ veins.

4. Buckling of the penile shaft in an erect or a semi-erect state is thought to cause _____.

5. Peyronie's disease affects _____ of men.

6. An increase in arterial inflow, smooth muscle relaxation in the corpora cavernosa, and an increase in venous resistance results in _____.

7. Patients with _____ may be more likely to develop Peyronie's disease due to increased risk of penile buckling and trauma, resulting in plaque formation.

8. _____ priapism results from impaired drainage of blood causing stasis of deoxygenated blood and compartment syndrome.

9. It is essential to differentiate between ischemic and nonischemic priapism because _____ is completely different.

10. A noninvasive method for assessing overall penile vascular health is the _____.

11. The methods used to obtain penile waveforms and pressures include CW Doppler or _____.

12. A pitfall of indirect, noninvasive evaluation of penile blood flow is that is does not provide specific _____ information regarding blood vessels of presence of plaques.

13. The typical transducer frequency used for penile duplex ultrasound is _____.

14. A preferred location to image the cavernosal arteries is at the _____ junction on the ventral aspect of the penis.

15. A potential complication from intracavernosal injection is _____, a prolonged erection without stimulation.

16. The primary diagnostic tool for the evaluation of erectile dysfunction due to vascular disease is _____ in the cavernosal artery.

17. Plaques within the tunica correspond anatomically to the _____ of the curvature on the penis.

18. Normal velocities in the cavernosal arteries postinjection are _____.

19. A EDV >5 cm/s in the cavernosal artery during peak erection is consistent with _____ dysfunction.

20. A venous velocity increase above 4 cm/s in the deep dorsal vein is associated with _____.

Short Answer

1. What are the typical indications for performance of ultrasound examination of the penis?

2. What are other causes of penile deformity besides Peyronie's disease?

3. What are the goals of a penile Doppler ultrasound study with intracavernosal injection?

IMAGE EVALUATION/PATHOLOGY

Review the images and answer the following questions.

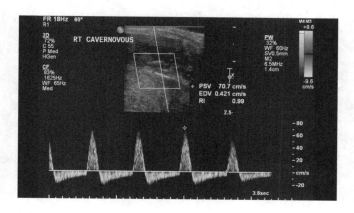

1. What is demonstrated in this cavernosal artery?

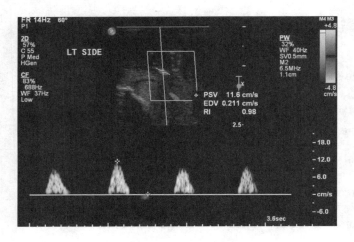

2. What is demonstrated in this cavernosal artery?

CASE STUDY

Review the information and answer the following questions.

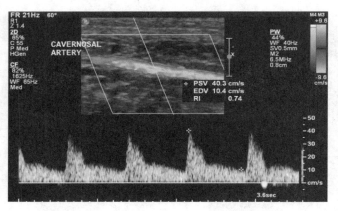

1. A patient presents to the vascular lab for evaluation of erectile dysfunction. The patient undergoes indirect testing and a brachial pressure of 136 mm Hg is obtained with a penile pressure of 68 mm Hg. What is the penile–brachial index? Is the index normal or abnormal? The patient also undergoes duplex ultrasound assessment. The above image was obtained during this evaluation. What is demonstrated in this image? What disease does this suggest?

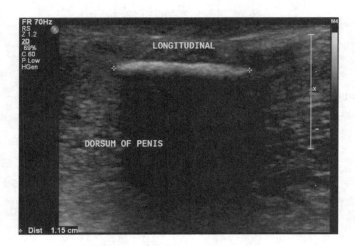

2. A patient presents to the vascular lab for evaluation of erectile dysfunction. During the duplex assessment, the above image was noted postinjection. Is this waveform normal or abnormal? Why? What does this waveform suggest regarding the patient's erectile dysfunction?

Vascular Applications of Ultrasound Contrast Agents

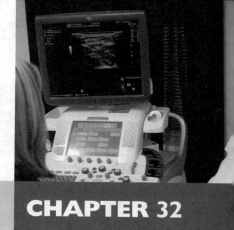

CHAPTER 32

REVIEW OF GLOSSARY TERMS

Matching

Match the key terms with their definitions.

KEY TERMS

1. _____ ultrasound contrast agent

2. _____ microbubbles

3. _____ contrast-enhanced sonography

DEFINITION

a. The use of medical ultrasound imaging after administration of an ultrasound contrast agent
b. Compositions that, after administration, alter the acoustic properties of body tissues, typically resulting in higher ultrasound signal reflectivity
c. Encapsulated gas-containing structures that are typically smaller than 8 microns in size

CHAPTER REVIEW

Multiple Choice

Complete each question by circling the best answer.

1. The "bubbles" used for ultrasound contrast are typically smaller than what?
   a. 2 microns
   b. 4 microns
   c. 6 microns
   d. 8 microns

2. For what reason are contrast agents approved for use in the United States?
   a. abdominal organ
   b. echocardiography
   c. peripheral vascular
   d. retroperitoneal

3. Which of the following is NOT a disadvantage of using saline as a contrast agent?
   a. persist through pulmonary circulation
   b. nonuniform in size
   c. relatively large size
   d. unstable or fragile

4. What is the microbubble shell in Definity?
   a. human serum albumin
   b. lipid
   c. galactose and palmitic acid
   d. phospholipid

5. Which of the following is NOT a characteristic of a viable contrast agent?
   a. nontoxic to a wide variety of patients
   b. microparticles that pass pulmonary capillary bed
   c. size greater than 8 microns
   d. stable to recirculate through CV system

6. How is the ultrasound contrast agent administered?
   a. oral
   b. intramuscular
   c. intravenous
   d. central line

7. Approximately how long will contrast administered in a bolus dose provide enhanced visualization?
   a. 2 minutes
   b. 4 minutes
   c. 8 minutes
   d. 12 minutes

8. Which of the following applications would be best suited for slow IV infusion of contrast agent?
   a. cardiac chamber opacification
   b. identification of large vessel wall
   c. identification of aneurysm
   d. organ perfusion

9. After the microbubbles are ruptured, how are the shell particles removed from the body?
   a. metabolized
   b. absorption
   c. excretion
   d. exhalation

10. Which type of UCA would best serve a patient/sonographer when the diagnosis is DVT and vessels are difficult to visualize?
    a. blood pool agent
    b. molecular imaging agent
    c. thrombus-specific agent
    d. tissue-specific agent

11. Which of the following is NOT an ultrasound system setting necessary for successful use of contrast agents?
    a. flash echo
    b. low mechanical index
    c. high acoustic output power
    d. harmonic imaging

12. Which of the following situations would most likely be enhanced with the use of contrast ultrasound agent?
    a. carotid with diagnostic level images
    b. deep vessels with luminal echogenicity
    c. vessels with slow flow identified by power Doppler
    d. postoperative complicated bypass surgery

13. In PAD, in which situation would using contrast agent improve the diagnostic quality of examination?
    a. atherosclerotic plaque on posterior vessel wall
    b. occlusion of the proximal femoral artery
    c. perfusion deficit of calf muscle
    d. DVT of popliteal vein

14. Which of the following does NOT limit sonographic visualization of intracranial vessels?

    a. acoustic windows

    b. high-velocity flow

    c. signal attenuation

    d. vessel branches

15. In which situation is duplex sonography least effective in the evaluation of organ transplant?

    a. postsurgical fluid collections

    b. urinary or bile obstructions

    c. blood flow to and from organ

    d. tissue perfusion

16. What is the most significant advantage to CES over repeated CT for evaluation of endovascular leaks?

    a. real-time blood flow assessment

    b. lack of ionizing radiation

    c. less chance of renal failure

    d. ability to detect leak flow

17. What would the use of contrast-enhanced ultrasound in the abdominal vasculature prove MOST helpful in?

    a. renal artery stent demonstrating laminar flow

    b. abdominal aortic aneurysm demonstrating true and false lumen

    c. turbulent blood flow through a TIPS

    d. competent endovascular graft of abdominal aorta

18. In a cardiac application, what would the use of a saline contrast study help diagnose?

    a. left-to-right shunting VSD

    b. patent ductus arteriosus

    c. left ventricular aneurysm

    d. patent foramen ovale

19. When assessing for vessel occlusion with contrast-enhanced sonography, what are the expected findings?

    a. vessel visualization distal to occlusion

    b. vessel visualization with no enhanced distal flow

    c. delayed vessel opacification

    d. visualization of flow "around" echogenic plaque in vessel

20. What would contrast-enhanced sonographic imaging in the cerebrovascular circulation prove helpful in?

    a. delineation of plaque ulceration

    b. assessment of functional lumen

    c. identification of string flow

    d. all the above

Fill-in-the-Blank

1. Ultrasound contrast agents alter the _____ of body tissues, resulting in higher signal reflectivity.

2. The use of contrast agents has been shown to _____ limitations of ultrasound imaging, which include contrast resolution on grayscale, slow blood flow, and small vessels.

3. When a vascular agent's microbubbles are ruptured or otherwise destroyed, the shell products are _____, and the gas is _____.

4. Tissue-specific agents must possess two unique characteristics: _____ for the targeted tissue and ability to alter that tissue's _____ appearance.

5. Tissue-specific UCAs target specific types of tissues with a predictable behavior, so they are considered _____.

6. Although blood pool agents help to better delineate the functional _____ of arteries and veins, they do not enhance the appearance of _____.

7. Thrombus-targeting UCAs have a therapeutic function by enhancing _____ when insonated.

8. _____ imaging is performed with the same transducers as used for conventional ultrasound and enhances the effectiveness of contrast agent visualization.

9. In harmonic imaging, the echoes from _____ microbubbles have a higher signal to noise ratio than conventional ultrasound imaging.

10. When contrast microbubbles are destroyed in an organ, the sonographer is able to observe _____ of the tissue.

11. UCAs allow for improved delineation of endocardial borders, assessment of regional wall motion, and detection of intracavitary thrombus in the field of _____.

12. Some of the main limitations in iliac vessel visualization that can be overcome with UCAs are overlying _____ and _____ vessels.

13. In peripheral artery disease evaluations of symptomatic patients, the two areas of improved visualization with CES are perfusion deficits and _____.

14. Contrast agents are most frequently administered via _____ extremity intravenous access site.

15. The use of contrast-enhanced sonography in the cerebrovascular circulation can be used to differentiate tight stenosis from _____.

16. Some investigators have compared _____ to tumors because of the requirement of nutrient-rich blood supply to grow.

17. Abdominal vascular applications of contrast-enhanced imaging include arterial and venous systems as well as abdominal _____ perfusion and masses.

18. A significant number of patients have anatomic variations of renal vasculature, including _____ renal arteries.

19. The enhancement capabilities of UCAs have been shown to have the ability to _____ nondiagnostic US examination.

20. Contrast agents available for use in the United States are _____, _____ and _____.

Short Answer

1. Describe clinical situations where using a bolus injection would be more beneficial than slow IV infusion.

2. What are the three types/mechanisms of contrast agents?

3. Overall, what can ultrasound contrast agents help in the detection of in the vascular system?

IMAGE EVALUATION/PATHOLOGY

Review the images and answer the following questions.

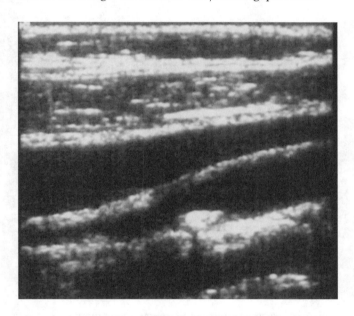

1. These images were taken from the mid-neck near the carotid bulb. What is demonstrated in these images? Is this clear from just the grayscale image?

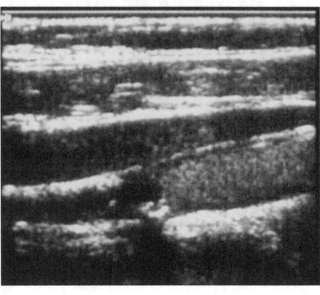

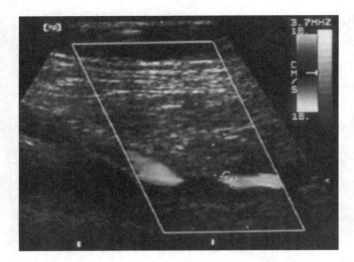

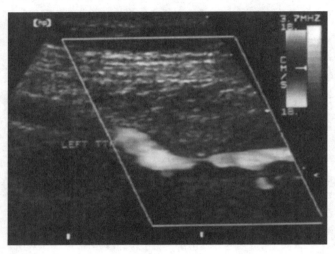

2. These images were obtained through the mid-calf. Describe the findings before and after contrast injection.

CASE STUDY

Review the information and answer the following questions.

1. A 67-year-old male patient with known peripheral vascular disease presents to the emergency department complaining of acute onset PAD symptoms in his right lower extremity. The patient was discharged just 3 days ago after undergoing surgical revascularization of the limb with new symptoms. If contrast-enhanced imaging were available, describe the potential sonographic findings in this patient.

2. A 57-year-old female with numerous cardiovascular risk factors presents for a cerebrovascular duplex examination. She has a left carotid bruit and has recently experienced visual disturbances in her right eye and left-sided weakness that have slowly resolved. What might you expect to see with and without the use of contrast-enhanced sonography?

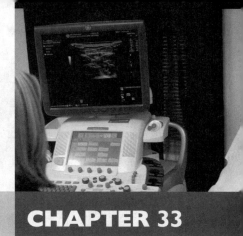

Complementary Vascular Imaging

REVIEW OF GLOSSARY TERMS

Matching

Match the key terms with their definitions.

KEY TERMS

1. _____ contrast

2. _____ enhancement

3. _____ subtraction

4. _____ reformat/reconstruction

5. _____ spatial resolution

DEFINITION

a. Alternate presentation of a digital image (i.e., three-dimensional volume rendered reconstruction)

b. Increase in image brightness within a vascular lumen after contrast injection

c. A pharmaceutic agent injected as part of an imaging test to distinguish vessels from nonvascular structures, and to highlight changes in size and shape of vessels

d. Ability of an imaging test to discriminate fine detail

e. Electronic manipulation of an image leaving only the contrast-enhanced structures visible

CHAPTER REVIEW

Multiple Choice

Complete each question by circling the best answer.

1. What is the gold standard for imaging evaluation of blood vessels?
   a. duplex sonography
   b. CT angiography
   c. MR angiography
   d. contrast arteriography

2. How does angiography generate images of vascular lumina?
   a. exposure to x-rays in a cross-sectional technique
   b. exposure to x-rays with vessels filled with iodinated contrast
   c. exposure to strong magnetic field with gadolinium contrast
   d. exposure to high-frequency sound waves without use of contrast

3. What technique is achieved by obtaining a mask image before injection of contrast and then a postinjection image is obtained of just the contrast filled vessels?
   a. CT angiography
   b. MR angiography
   c. digital subtraction angiography
   d. color Duplex imaging

4. Which modality allows digital reconstruction of images into three-dimensional images?
   a. duplex sonography
   b. MRA
   c. DSA
   d. CTA

5. What is the typical rate of contrast injection for CTA?
   a. 1 to 2 mL/s
   b. 3 to 5 mL/s
   c. 5 to 7 mL/s
   d. 7 to 10 mL/s

6. Which of the following is a limitation of CTA when trying to determine stenosis versus occlusion, especially in small vessels?
   a. intimal calcification
   b. patient body habitus
   c. low-flow state
   d. extravasation of contrast

7. What is a benefit of MRA compared to CTA?
   a. does not require contrast
   b. not motion dependent
   c. cannot be used in patients with metallic implants
   d. no exposure to ionizing radiation

8. When using contrast injections with either CT or MR, what must the patient do when images need to be acquired?
   a. turn on their side
   b. hold their breath
   c. perform a Valsalva maneuver
   d. perform a series of cognitive tasks

9. Where is MRA the least accurate?
   a. internal carotid artery
   b. peripheral arteries
   c. visceral vessels
   d. peripheral veins

10. What is the typically use of DSA in the cerebrovascular system?
    a. diagnostic purposes
    b. guidance of therapeutic interventions
    c. surveillance after intervention
    d. DSA no longer used in this system

11. Which modality is particularly useful in demonstrating vascular anomalies, collateral pathways, and soft tissues surrounding the vasculature?
    a. CTA
    b. MRA
    c. duplex sonography
    d. DSA

12. Which modality is better suited for patients with iodine allergies or who are diabetics?
    a. CTA
    b. MRA
    c. duplex sonography
    d. DSA

13. Which modality is the first-line modality for diagnosis of venous thrombosis?
    a. CTA
    b. MRA
    c. duplex sonography
    d. DSA

14. Which modality can be used in pregnant patients without contrast administration to visualize pelvic veins?
    a. MRV
    b. CTV
    c. contrast venography
    d. CT without contrast

15. Which modality is generally NOT recommended to be used in the setting of acute trauma?
    a. CTA
    b. DSA
    c. MRA
    d. duplex sonography

Fill-in-the-Blank

1. Digital subtraction angiography is a(n) _____ technique and, as a result, usually requires multiple projections to adequately display arterial lesions.

2. _____ are configured with an x-ray source emitting a fan-shaped beam, mounted on a rotating ring opposite an arc of x-ray detectors.

3. CTA has essentially replaced _____ for the diagnosis of pulmonary embolism.

4. Because of the frequency of CT performance, risk of radiation-induced _____ is a concern.

5. The basis of MR images is _____ energy from proton movement from application of magnetic gradients.

6. Noncontrast MRA uses _____ method to visualize blood vessels.

7. Stents, filters, and other vascular implants generate artifacts on MRA that can render the study _____.

8. Patients with poor renal function are at risk for the development of nephrogenic systemic fibrosis after exposure to gadolinium-based contrast agents especially with glomerular filtration rates of _____.

9. CT and MR allow for visualization of vessel wall and intimal plaque, whereas DSA only depicts the _____.

10. The cross-sectional nature of CT and MR allows for improved characterization of _____ vessel narrowing over projectional DSA images.

11. _____ are especially useful with central veins, where sonographic access is limited.

12. The gold standard for the evaluation of aortic dissection and aortic aneurysm prior to intervention is _____.

13. _____ is not useful after renal artery stenting as a result of artifacts caused by the stent.

14. While many modalities are useful to demonstrate the origins of mesenteric vessels, _____ is necessary to depict smaller branch vessels that are more often involved in embolic disease and vasculitis.

15. The initial test after trauma is typically _____ owing to its ability to visualize soft tissue as well as vascular structures.

Short Answer

1. What are the limitations and contraindications of digital subtraction angiography?

2. How do CT and MR compare regarding applications and limitations?

IMAGE EVALUATION/PATHOLOGY

Review the images and answer the following questions.

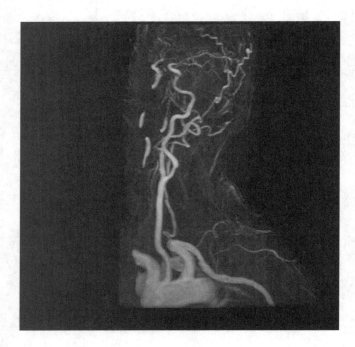

1. What is demonstrated in this MRA?

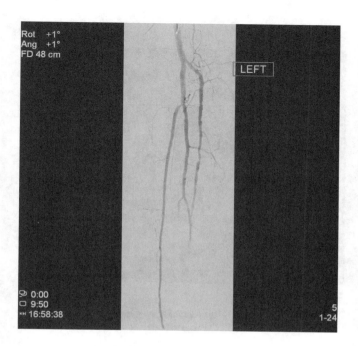

2. What is demonstrated in this DSA image of the infrapopliteal circulation?

3. What is demonstrated in this coronal MRV?

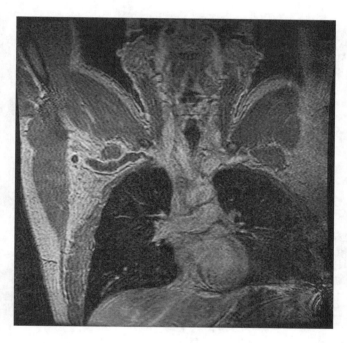

4. What is demonstrated in this CTA?

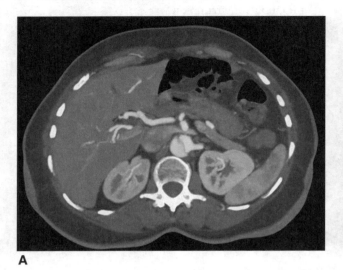

A

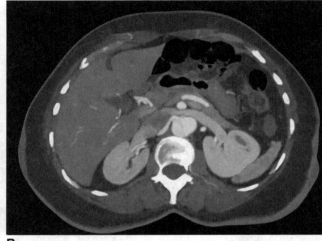

B

CASE STUDY

1. A 66-year-old male patient underwent duplex sonography for evaluation of renal artery stenosis. On the duplex examination, indirect evidence of renal artery stenosis was obtained from the renal hilum; however, the main renal arteries were not adequately visualized. Which imaging modality would most likely be used next to confirm the diagnosis of renal artery stenosis?

2. A visibly agitated patient presents for imaging evaluation for peripheral arterial disease. This patient has a history of trauma as well as evidence of peripheral arterial disease. What is the main purpose of vascular diagnosis for the lower extremities? Which imaging would be most likely initially used in this patient given his history?

Quality Assurance Statistics

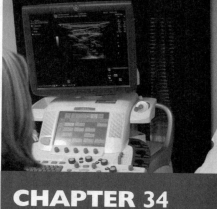

REVIEW OF GLOSSARY TERMS

Matching

Match the key terms with their definitions.

KEY TERMS

1. _____ gold standard

2. _____ accuracy

3. _____ sensitivity

4. _____ specificity

5. _____ positive predictive value

6. _____ negative predictive value

7. _____ peer review

DEFINITION

a. The ability of a test to correctly identify a normal result
b. The proportion of patients with positive test results that are correctly identified
c. The overall percentage of correct results
d. The proportion of negative test results when there is no underlying disease present
e. The ability of a test to detect disease
f. A well-established and reliable testing parameter, which for vascular disease is often angiography
g. The evaluation of one's work by other experts in the same field

CHAPTER REVIEW

Multiple Choice

Complete each question by circling the best answer.

1. In vascular testing, what is typically considered to be the gold standard?
   a. computed tomography
   b. magnetic resonance imaging
   c. angiography
   d. duplex ultrasound

2. What is the identification of a 50% to 79% stenosis of the internal carotid artery and a 60% stenosis by angiography an example of?
   a. true positive
   b. true negative
   c. false positive
   d. false negative

3. Upon ultrasound evaluation, DVT is found in the popliteal vein; however, venography demonstrates a widely patent vessel. What is this an example of?
   a. true positive
   b. true negative
   c. false positive
   d. false negative

4. During duplex assessment of the abdominal aorta, the aorta measures <2.0 cm, which is confirmed by angiography. What is this an example of?
   a. true positive
   b. true negative
   c. false positive
   d. false negative

5. Duplex evaluation of the superior mesenteric artery demonstrated velocities of 150 cm/s. Angiography demonstrated a 70% stenosis in the same vessel. What is this an example of?
   a. true positive
   b. true negative
   c. false positive
   d. false negative

6. Which of the following is NOT likely to occur if false-positive results are indicated by the duplex ultrasound examination?
   a. unnecessary treatment
   b. lack of treatment when treatment is needed
   c. unnecessary stress to the patient
   d. repeat examinations

7. Which of the following would have the highest accuracy?
   a. 25 true positives and 30 true negatives out of 100 exams
   b. 20 true positives and 10 true negatives out of 100 exams
   c. 50 true positives and 5 true negatives out of 100 exams
   d. 10 true positives and 75 true negatives out of 100 exams

8. An increase in which of the following results would increase the sensitivity of an exam?
   a. false positive
   b. false negative
   c. true positive
   d. true negative

9. Which results are needed to improve specificity?
   a. true negatives
   b. true positives
   c. false negatives
   d. false positives

10. What is the consistency of obtaining similar results under similar circumstances?
    a. accuracy
    b. sensitivity
    c. reliability
    d. specificity

11. Which of the following would an increase in the number of false-positive results have an impact on?
    a. positive predictive value and negative predictive value
    b. positive predictive value and specificity
    c. negative predictive value and sensitivity
    d. positive predictive value and sensitivity

12. After statistical analysis, a test was found to have a sensitivity of 92% and a specificity of 84%. Which of the following could represent the overall accuracy?
    a. 95%
    b. 82%
    c. 89%
    d. cannot be determined

13. If a test has a negative predictive value of 50%, how sure can you be that your test results are negative?
    a. extremely
    b. moderately
    c. equivocal
    d. not sure at all

14. In general, if the sensitivity of a test increases, what will happen to the specificity of the test?
    a. also increases
    b. decreases
    c. remains the same
    d. cannot be determined

15. Which of the following parameters would an increase in the number of false negative results impact?
    a. negative predictive value and sensitivity
    b. positive predicative value and sensitivity
    c. sensitivity and specificity
    d. negative predictive value and specificity

Fill-in-the-Blank

1. _____ refers to a program for the systematic monitoring and evaluation of the various aspects of vascular testing to ensure that standards of quality are being met.

2. _____ is the science of making effective use of numerical data relating to groups of individuals or experiments.

3. A _____ is used to compare one form of a newer diagnostic test with another that is well established and reliable.

4. _____ are the number of studies performed by ultrasound, which state that disease is present and the gold standard agrees with the ultrasound findings.

5. _____ are the number of studies performed by ultrasound, which state that disease is not present and are also reported as negative by the gold standard.

6. Studies that are reported positive by ultrasound but are found to be negative by the gold standard are known as _____.

7. If a study is normal on ultrasound but the gold standard identifies disease, it is an example of a _____.

8. Accuracy is calculated as the _____ number of correct tests _____ by the total number of all tests.

9. _____ is calculated by taking the true positive results and dividing these by all positive results as determined by the gold standard.

10. Dividing the number of true negatives by all the negative results as identified by the gold standard results in the _____ of the test.

11. A vascular laboratory that has an overall accuracy of 96% over an average of 5 years would be said to be _____.

12. _____ is calculated as the number of true positives divided by all the positive studies.

13. True negatives divided by all studies determined to be negative results in the _____.

14. In a chi-square analysis, boxes A and B are used to determine _____, whereas boxes C and D are used to determine _____.

15. In a chi-square analysis, boxes A and C are used to determine _____, whereas boxes B and D are used to determine _____.

Short Answer

1. As the technical director of the vascular laboratory, you are asked to complete a statistical analysis of a particular duplex test. You collect the following data:

   150 test results that were negative both by duplex and angiography

   75 test results that were positive both by duplex and angiography

   15 test results that were positive by duplex but negative by angiography

   10 test results that were negative by duplex but positive by angiography

   What are the sensitivity, specificity, positive predictive value, negative predictive value, and overall accuracy for this test?

2. In examining another test, you collect the following data: 500 total tests of which 300 were negative. Of the negative tests, 200 agreed with the gold standard. Of the positive tests, 100 agreed with the gold standard. What are the sensitivity, specificity, positive predictive value, negative predictive value, and overall accuracy of this test? How would you interpret these results?